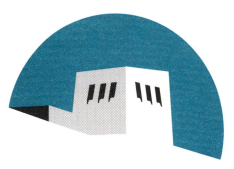

Diabetes Annual 2002

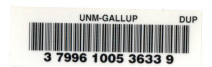

Diabetes Annual 2002

Edited by

Anthony H Barnett MD FRCP

Professor of Medicine and Consultant Physician
Department of Medicine/Diabetes/Endocrinology
Birmingham Heartlands Hospital
Birmingham, UK

MARTIN DUNITZ

First published in the United Kingdom in 2002
by Martin Dunitz Ltd, The Livery House, 7–9 Pratt Street, London NW1 0AE

Tel.:   +44 (0) 20 7482 2202
Fax: +44 (0) 20 7267 0159
E-mail: info@dunitz.co.uk
Website: http://www.dunitz.co.uk

A CIP record for this book is available from the British Library.

ISBN 1 84184 038 6

Distributed in the USA by
Fulfilment Center
Taylor & Francis
7625 Empire Drive
Florence, KY 41042, USA
Toll Free Tel: 1-800-634-7064
E-mail: cserve@routledge_ny.com

Distributed in Canada by
Taylor & Francis
74 Rolark Drive
Scarborough
Ontario M1R 4G2, Canada
Toll Free Tel: 1-877-226-2237
E-mail: tal_fran@istar.ca

Distributed in the rest of the world by
ITPS Limited
Cheriton House
North Way, Andover
Hampshire SP10 5BE, UK
Tel: +44 (0)1264 332424
E-mail: reception@itps.co.uk

Composition by Wearset Ltd, Boldon, Tyne and Wear

Printed and bound in Great Britain by Biddles Ltd, Guildford and King's Lynn

Contents

List of contributors

William D Alexander FRCP
Diabetes Unit, Western General
Hospital, Edinburgh, UK.

Shahid Ali MB PhD
Centre for Research in Primary Care,
Leeds, UK.

Amit Allahabadia MD
Department of Diabetes and
Endocrinology, Northern General
Hospital, Sheffield, UK.

Antonella Caselli MD
Joslin–Beth Israel Deaconess Foot
Center and Microcirculation Laboratory,
Department of Surgery, Beth-Israel
Deaconess Medical Center; Harvard
Medical School, Boston MA, USA.

Mark E Cooper PhD MD
Department of Medicine, University of
Melbourne, Austin & Repatriation
Medical Centre, West Heidelberg,
Victoria, Australia.

Paul M Dodson MD FRCP FRCOphth
Department of Diabetes, University of
Birmingham, Birmingham Heartlands
Hospital, Birmingham, UK.

Panayiotis A Economides MD
Joslin Diabetes Center and Division of
Endocrinology, Beth Israel Deaconess
Medical Center, Harvard Medical
School, Boston MA, USA.

Brian M Frier MD FRCPE
Department of Diabetes, Royal
Infirmary, Edinburgh, UK.

Simon R Heller DM FRCP
University of Sheffield, Northern
General Hospital, Sheffield, UK.

Sudhesh Kumar MD FRCP
Department of Diabetes and
Endocrinology, Birmingham Heartlands
Hospital, Birmingham, UK.

Elaine Murphy MSc MRCPI
Department of Metabolic Medicine,
Imperial College School of Medicine,
Hammersmith Hospital, London, UK.

John J Nolan FRCPI
Metabolic Research Unit, Department
of Endocrinology, St James's Hospital,
Dublin, Ireland.

Matthew D Oldfield MD
Department of Medicine, University of
Melbourne, Austin & Repatriation
Medical Centre, West Heidelberg,
Victoria, Australia.

Andrew J Sommerfield MB MRCP (UK)
Department of Diabetes, Royal
Infirmary of Edinburgh, Edinburgh, UK.

Aristidis Veves MD DSc
Joslin–Beth Israel Deaconess Foot
Center and Microcirculation Laboratory,
Department of Surgery, Beth-Israel
Deaconess Medical Center; Harvard
Medical School, Boston MA, USA.

Rhys Williams
Nuffield Institute for Health, Leeds, UK.

Preface

We are presently facing a global epidemic of diabetes which is set to get much worse within the next 20 years. In recent decades the numbers of Type 2 diabetic patients have, in particular, increased and will continue to increase exponentially. The reasons for this relate in part to an ageing population, but mainly to the great increase in rates of obesity and sedentary lifestyle which has occurred in many countries of the world in recent years. Type 2 diabetes now accounts for around 95% of all cases worldwide. In addition, the long-term complications of diabetes cause much morbidity and mortality; by far the most important of these complications is cardiovascular disease. This will kill over 75% of all diabetic patients, many prematurely, and has led to a re-definition of Type 2 diabetes as a condition of premature cardiovascular disease.

Coincident with the increasing numbers of diabetic patients, there have also been significant advances in our understanding of the pathophysiology of the condition and a firm evidence base has developed for management of cardiovascular risk factors which so commonly co-occur in the same patient. There have also been major developments in new therapies both for the management of diabetes and its complications. These many advances in both the understanding of the condition and new therapies are the major reasons for publication of the 2002 issue of the *Diabetes Annual*. Each chapter has been written by an expert (or experts) in their field. The first chapter covers epidemiology, classification and new diagnostic criteria as a lead into subsequent chapters which cover the relationship between diabetes, obesity and cardiovascular disease and further consideration of the evidence base for treatment of hypertension in diabetes, together with prevention and treatment of microvascular disease. This is followed by chapters on hypoglycaemia and then new therapies, including the thiazolidinediones and insulin analogues. The difficult issue of erectile dysfunction is then considered, followed finally by a review of new therapies for the treatment of diabetic neuropathy.

This book is written for a specialist audience and should be of interest to diabetologists, diabetologists in training, diabetes nurse educators and GPs with a special interest. I hope that the result is a highly readable, interesting, practical and relevant publication.

1

Diabetes: epidemiology, classification and new diagnostic criteria – implications for clinical practice?

Rhys Williams and Shahid Ali

Definition and classification of diabetes – a developing understanding

The current prevalence of Type 1 and Type 2 diabetes is now well documented for many of the world's regions and countries. Fundamental to this documentation are the standardization of diagnostic criteria for diabetes and related conditions, the classification of the different subtypes of diabetes and the standardization of methods for the conduct of population-based prevalence studies.

The American Diabetes Association (ADA)[1] and the World Health Organization (WHO)[2] have recently suggested revisions of the diagnostic criteria for diabetes and the related conditions of impaired glucose tolerance (IGT) and impaired fasting glucose (IFG). These ADA and WHO recommendations are similar but not, unfortunately, identical. `

The main similarity is a revision, downwards (compared with previous WHO criteria),[3] of the minimum blood glucose concentration necessary for the diagnosis of diabetes. Such periodic revisions of threshold values are necessary in the light of accumulating evidence on the long-term significance of given blood glucose levels. The minimum fasting blood glucose concentration necessary for the diagnosis of diabetes is now recommended to be 7.0mmol/l (120mg/dl) compared with the previous 7.8mmol/l (140mg/dl).

One of the important differences between ADA and WHO relates to the method of testing for diabetes. ADA advocates a move away from the 2 hour oral glucose tolerance test (OGTT) and a reliance, instead, on measuring the fasting blood glucose alone; WHO is more supportive of the continuing use of the OGTT. The emphasis on IFG as a category of abnormal glucose tolerance is related to the reliance on the fasting blood glucose concentration alone; IGT cannot be diagnosed without both fasting and 2 hour values.

Table 1.1 Classification of diabetes - adapted from ADA.[1]

Type 1 diabetes	β-cell destruction, usually leading to absolute insulin deficiency
Type 2 diabetes	May range from predominantly insulin resistance with relative insulin deficiency to a predominantly secretory defect with insulin resistance

Other specific types

- Genetic defects of β-cell function [e.g. chromosome 7, glucokinase (formerly MODY2)]
- Genetic defects in insulin action (e.g. leprechaunism)
- Diseases of the exocrine pancreas (e.g. pancreatitis)
- Endocrinopathies (e.g. acromegaly)
- Drug or chemical induced diabetes (e.g. caused by thiazides)
- Infections (e.g. congenital rubella)
- Uncommon forms of immune-mediated diabetes (e.g. due to anti-insulin antibodies)
- Other genetic syndromes sometimes associated with diabetes (e.g. Down's syndrome)

Gestational diabetes mellitus

The classification system now advocated is shown in Table 1.1. Both ADA and WHO favour a move away from the previous terms of insulin-dependent diabetes (mellitus) (IDD or IDDM) and non-insulin-dependent diabetes (mellitus) (NIDD or NIDDM) to an aetiological classification using the terms Type 1 and Type 2 diabetes, respectively, instead. The Type 1 process predominantly consists of pancreatic β-cell destruction leading to a state of insulin deficiency. The Type 2 process is viewed as progressing from an initial state dominated by insulin resistance to one in which relative insulin deficiency predominates as a result of an insulin secretory defect. Adopting these new terms will reduce the confusion generated by the fact that some patients who are said to have NIDD may have insulin-treated diabetes. As more attention is given to striving for near-normal levels of glycaemic control, more and more patients with Type 2 diabetes are likely to be treated with insulin.

Understanding of the genetic predisposition of Type 1 diabetes is now fairly well advanced. Both genetic predisposition and environmental factors play a part in its aetiology. The locus named IDDM1,[4] situated on the short arm of chromosome 6, is the major genetic determinant with a number of others, scattered throughout the genome, playing less significant roles. As ADA and WHO advocate a move away from the term IDDM it is unfortunate that it should continue in use in describing these loci.

On the other hand, Type 2 diabetes is still something of a geneticists nightmare. The most well characterized subtype of Type 2 diabetes – maturity onset diabetes of the young (MODY) – is itself subdivided into a number of separately identifiable conditions (e.g. MODY1, MODY2, etc.) (see Table 1.1). Each of these conditions is dominantly inherited with a specific metabolic lesion; however, some do and some do not have the characteristic originally ascribed to MODY (or Mason-type diabetes as it was then known), i.e. freedom from the microvascular complications of diabetes. Apart from this, and some knowledge about the genetics and metabolic basis of a small fraction of the remainder of type 2 diabetes, knowledge of the genetics of the c. 80% of diabetes cases this represents is rudimentary.

The clear and absolute aetiological and genetic distinction between Type 1 and Type 2 diabetes, once regarded as a basic tenet, is now less strongly advocated than before. An illustration of this is latent autoimmune diabetes in adults (LADA), as what turns out, eventually, to be Type 1 diabetes may masquerade, in its early stages, as Type 2 diabetes.[5] This subtype of diabetes is associated, as is true Type 1 diabetes, with circulating antibodies to glutamic acid decarboxylase (GAD).[6]

Occurrence (incidence and prevalence) of diabetes – the current and future global scene

Amos et al.[7] and King et al.[8] have published estimates of the prevalence of diabetes in a large number of countries. More recently, the International Diabetes Federation (IDF) has collated updated estimates of some of these data.[9] Using this IDF publication as its source, Table 1.2 lists, for illustration, the countries with the highest and lowest percentage prevalence estimates in each of the IDF's regions. Prevalence is expressed both as the proportion of the population estimated to have diabetes (diagnosed and previously undiagnosed) and the estimated absolute number of people affected in the country.

Diabetes in the People's Republic of China provides a useful example of the need to consider both proportional and absolute prevalence when judging the extent of a national burden resulting from diabetes. Although mainland China is the country with the lowest proportional prevalence (2.7%) in its IDF region (Western Pacific), it has an estimated 22.5 million people with diabetes, more than any other country except India which, with a prevalence of 5.8%, has an estimated 32.7 million people affected. These prevalences are increasing, as in most other countries, although in a few the prevalence may be fairly static, but no country has so far been reported as having a declining prevalence of diabetes.

These same sources have also published predictions of future prevalence, as compared to Amos et al.'s that static projections, i.e. the latter

Table 1.2 Estimates of the prevalence of diabetes in adults (aged 20–79) in IDF regions for the year 2000 (adapted from IDF[9])

IDF Region*	Country	Prevalence (%)[†]	Number of people with diabetes
Africa			
Highest	South Africa	4.0	886,000
Lowest	Gambia	0.3	2200
EMME[‡]			
Highest	Bahrain	14.8	56,300
Lowest	Morocco	2.4	384,900
Europe			
Highest	Israel	7.2	273,700
Lowest	Iceland	1.9	3600
North America			
Highest	Barbados	13.2	24,200
Lowest	Guyana	3.1	16,000
South and Central America			
Highest	Netherlands Antilles	10.3	14,700
Lowest	Guatemala	2.9	148,900
	Panama	2.9	48,200
South East Asia			
Highest	Mauritius	15.0	112,600
Lowest	Sri Lanka	2.9	335,400
Western Pacific			
Highest	Papua New Guinea	15.5	378,300
Lowest	People's Republic of China	2.7	22,564,800

* Highest and lowest prevalence estimates are given but these are for all age groups or an adult age group other than those aged 20–79.
†Previously diagnosed and undiagnosed diabetes, the latter detected by the 2 hour oral glucose tolerance test (Gambia) or fasting blood glucose (Morocco), classified according to WHO criteria.[3]
‡Eastern Mediterranean and Middle East.

assumes constant age- and sex-specific incidence rates for diabetes and take into account only projected demographic changes. King et al.'s[8] projections have taken these demographic changes into account and also predictions of the future extent of urbanization. This phenomenon, particularly in developing countries, is likely to increase prevalence as a result of decreased physical activity and increased energy density of the diet.

There are few published dynamic predictions of future trends in diabetes prevalence. These are predictions that take into account, as well as changing demography, the likelihood that age- and sex-specific incidence rates will increase as the prevalence of risk markers changes.[10] Ruwaard et al.'s[11] predictions for the Netherlands suggest that, taking these dynamic elements into account, the predicted prevalence of diabetes in that country for 2005 is 2.1% rather than 1.6% of the population as predicted by their static model, using the same baseline prevalences, in both predictions.

An increase in the prevalence of diabetes from one year (1998) to the next has been documented in the USA by Mokdad et al.[12] Using data from the Behavioral Risk Factor Surveillance System, these authors reported that the overall prevalence of diabetes in adults increased from 6.5 ± 0.11% standard error of the mean (SEM) in 1998 to 6.9 ± 0.12% in 1999. There was a particularly striking increase in men (5.5 ± 0.15% to 6.0 ± 0.17%), in those of African-American descent (8.9 ± 0.39% to 9.9 ± 0.42%) and those with university level qualifications (4.4 ± 0.17% to 5.1 ± 0.19%). There increases were attributed to the rapid rise in obesity in the US population. The same group of researchers previously reported a rise in the prevalence of obesity [body mass index (BMI) $\rightarrow$ 30kg/m^2] from 12.0 to 17.9% in 1998.[13]

Epidemiological changes are not confined to Type 2 diabetes. Most population-based registers of Type 1 diabetes in children report significant increases in incidence with time. Although later years are likely to have seen increasingly complete ascertainment of cases, the reported rise in incidence is well accepted as a real phenomenon, although the reasons for it are still not understood. For example, in the UK, in the county of Yorkshire, a rise in incidence is reported for all age groups of children (0–4, 5–9 and 10–14 years of age) over the years from 1978 to 1998.[14] The mean annual increases in incidence are reported to be 2.5, 2.2 and 3.0% in each age group, respectively with an incidence of 26.6 per 100,000 children per year projected for 2005 and 30.2 per 100,000 for 2010 (compared with 15.5 in 1998). Absolute numbers of new cases in Yorkshire's total population of c. 700,000 children, are projected to increase from 110 cases per year in 1998 to 211 in 2010 if these predictions are fulfilled.

Further confirmation of this rising trend in incidence, but emphasizing that the phenomenon is most marked in younger children (those under 5 years of age), comes from Switzerland.[15] Using data collected from 434 girls and 507 boys in a nationwide questionnaire survey begun in 1991, these authors described a rise in incidence (for children between the ages of 0 and 14 from 7.8 per 100,000 per year to over 10.6 per 100,000 per year. This rise was the result of a more than fourfold increase in incidence (from 2.4 per 100,000 per year to 10.5 per 100,000 per year) in the 0–4-years-old age group, with increases in other age groups which did not reach statistical significance.

Of particular public health concern at present is the realization that lifestyle changes are beginning to transform Type 2 diabetes from a largely adult disorder into one also affecting teenagers[16] and children below the age of 10.[17] ADA considered this trend serious enough to issue a consensus statement on the identification, treatment and prevention of Type 2 diabetes in children.[18] Concern about the trend has also been expressed in the UK, e.g. a recent case series report from Birmingham in the West Midlands describes eight girls, between the ages of nine and 16, recently diagnosed as having Type 2 diabetes.[19] All were overweight 141–209% over their predicted weight for height, all had a family history of diabetes in at least two generations (though these were not MODY families) and all were of Pakistani, Indian or Arabic origin. They were initially treated with dietary modification, with oral hypoglycaemic agents added in seven cases; two were subsequently treated with insulin.

Implications for clinical practice of increasing prevalence and incidence, younger age at onset and new diagnostic criteria

The above discussion places into context the rising prevalence of diabetes globally. It also places a special emphasis on the lowered age of onset of Type 2 diabetes, a phenomenon that will clearly have an adverse impact on the future incidence and prevalence of complications. The rising prevalence both of Type 1 and Type 2 diabetes will have significant clinical implications for both primary and secondary care. These trends of increased numbers of people with diabetes being diagnosed early is likely to continue and then reach a steady state at some point in the future as the pool of individuals who are genetically predisposed becomes saturated.

The increasing understanding of the genetics of Type 1 diabetes may soon enable a prediction to be made of when and at what level of prevalence this saturation will occur. Conversely, the current knowledge of the genetics of Type 2 diabetes is so inadequate that there is no way of making accurate predictions, and it is this type of diabetes that impacts most on public health and clinical practice. International comparisons suggest, however, that the prevalence of Type 2 diabetes is likely to rise considerably from the 2–10% range currently seen in most countries.

A true rise in prevalence resulting from changes in lifestyle will be compounded by the impact on prevalence of recent changes in diagnostic criteria. Since, as a result of the ADA and WHO revisions described above, a person will be considered to have diabetes at a lower level of fasting blood glucose, this is likely to mean an overall rise in the number of people diagnosed with diabetes. However, the impact that these changes make will differ depending on the balance of fasting hyperglycaemia and postprandial hyperglycaemia present in any given population at any one time.

The lowering of the critical level of blood glucose in these recent recommendations, as stated above, is coupled with a shift away from the use of the 2 hour postglucose level in combination with the fasting level. Thus, in populations with diabetes predominantly resulting from postprandial hyperglycaemia, the prevalence may actually fall as a result of this abnormality being undetected. An example of this can be seen in the North American study of people between the ages of 40 and 74 described in the ADA Expert Committee Report,[1] in which analysis using the new ADA criteria led to a reduction in overall prevalence in this age group from 6.3 to 4.3%.

In contrast, in populations with diabetes predominantly resulting from fasting hyperglycaemia, a rise in prevalence will be seen when these criteria are introduced. Thus, Unwin et al.,[20] studying a population between the ages of 25 and 74 living in northeast England, found that the overall prevalence of diabetes increased from 4.8 to 7.1% in Caucasians, from 4.7 to 6.2% in people of Chinese origin and from 20.1 to 21.4% in people of South Asian origin when the recent ADA criteria were used for comparison with WHO criteria.[3]

Davies et al.[21] investigated the impact of the new criteria on the diagnosis of diabetes and other forms of abnormal glucose metabolism in people with symptoms of diabetes. Theirs was a retrospective analysis of 154 consecutive OGTT carried out on non-pregnant adults referred because of symptoms suggestive of diabetes. The results of the OGTT were analysed on the basis of 1985 WHO criteria (in use when the tests were carried out), the newly published ADA criteria and WHO criteria then advocated for consultation: the results are summarized in Table 1.3. On the basis of these results, the authors advocate use of the revised WHO criteria rather than ADA criteria, which seems sensible for a number of reasons, particularly the fact that use of ADA criteria eliminates the ability to identify those patients with IGT. IGT is a condition known for some time to increase risk, in terms of morbidity, from cardiovascular disease[22] and progression to diabetes, and is also known to have different characteristics compared with IFG.[23] The clinical significance of IFG, on the other hand, is virtually unknown but nothing is lost by adopting WHO criteria, since they can identify both IFG and IGT.

The impact on clinical practice of changes in the epidemiology of diabetes and revisions in diagnostic criteria will differ considerably from country to country, e.g. the susceptibility of populations to Type1 and Type 2 diabetes, the organization of health-care systems and the financial resources that can be devoted to health care and prevention will all have some affect. Three very different counties have been selected to illustrate these differences – Finland, Bangladesh and the UK. Of these, the UK will be described in most detail because of the authors' first-hand knowledge of public health and clinical practice in that country. First, however, the contrasting situations in Finland and Bangladesh will be described and discussed.

Table 1.3 Comparison of the diagnostic classification of 154 2 hour oral glucose tolerance tests of people with symptoms suggestive of diabetes, using 1985 WHO criteria, ADA criteria and 1997 WHO criteria (adapted from Davies et al.[21])

Criteria and ethnic group	Diabetes	Impaired glucose tolerance	Impaired fasting glucose	Normal
1985 WHO				
Caucasian	18 (12%)	22 (14%)	NG	25 (16%)
Asian	51 (33%)	26 (17%)	NG	12 (8%)
Total	69 (45%)	48* (31%)	4 (3%)	37[†] (24%)
1997 ADA				
Caucasian	15 (10%)	NA	5 (3%)	45 (29%)
Asian	36 (23%)	NA	12 (8%)	41 (27%)
Total	51 (33%)	NA	17 (11%)	86 (56%)
1998 WHO				
Caucasian	22 (14%)	18 (12%)	NG	25 (16%)
Asian	52 (34%)	25 (16%)	NG	12 (8%)
Total	74 (48%)	43* (28%)	4 (3%)	37 (24%)

*Including four people also with impaired fasting glucose.
†Text of reference 21 gives 33, table above gives 37 – the latter is correct.
NA, not applicable (because a 2 hour sample is required to classify people as having impaired glucose tolerance and the 1997 ADA criteria do not advocate a 2 hour sample being taken); NG, = not given in reference 21.

Finland

Finland occupies a particularly important place in the epidemiology of Type 1 diabetes. It has long-established, comprehensive, population-based registers of childhood diabetes and, largely as a result of these registers, is well known as having, currently, the highest incidence rates for childhood diabetes recorded anywhere in the world. The IDF's Diabetes Atlas 2000 records an annual incidence of diabetes in children (0–14 years of age) of 45.0 per 100,000, which compares with an incidence of 5.0 per 100,000 in Bangladesh and 18.0 per 100,000 in the UK.[9]

The overall prevalence of diabetes (Type 1 and Type 2, previously diagnosed and newly detected) in adults between the ages of 45 and 64 in Finland is 5.5%.[24] Thus, the challenge to Finnish health services includes Type 2 as well as Type 1 diabetes.

Organized care for people with diabetes in Finland originates from the plan published, in 1976, by the State Diabetes Committee; this, and the situation current in the early 1980s, is described in detail by Aro.[25] The characteristics of the system at that time were organization on a regional scale, designated diabetes clinics at local health centres, and a key role for the diabetes nurse and the wider team in running local clinics, evaluating patient needs and conducting patient education. These characteristics, particularly local access, were seen as essential for a scattered population with relatively long distances to travel in order to access health care.

A more recent assessment of the state of diabetes care in Finland[26] emphasizes the fact that, despite this long-standing interest and emphasis on organized diabetes care, only 13% of a sample of just under 900 people with diabetes examined had good metabolic control and 25% had poor control [defined as glycated haemoglobin (HbA$_{1c}$) levels of <7.0% and $\rightarrow$ 10.0%, respectively]. Significant regional variation in standards of care were described and hospital use by people with diabetes was high, as compared with the general Finnish population and with international levels of hospital usage. This level of usage has considerable resource consequences for the health services. Important conclusions of this report, given predictions of an increase in the prevalence of Type 2 diabetes affecting Finland in common with all European countries, were that cooperation between primary care and secondary care should be improved, educational activities strengthened and insulin use among people with Type 2 diabetes promoted.

Bangladesh

One of the many ways in which Bangladesh and Finland differ is the contrast between the distributed, community based approach to diabetes care in the latter and the centralized approach taken in the former. As the diabetes epidemic develops in Bangladesh, however, this initially centralized approach is being expanded to accommodate the larger numbers of people with diabetes who need diagnosis, treatment and long-term surveillance.

Bangladesh is one of the poorest countries in the world. It has recognized diabetes as a significant health problem since 1956, when the vision of a group of social workers, philanthropists, physicians and civil servants, led by Professor M Ibrahim, founded the Diabetic Association of Bangladesh.[27] Since then, the service delivered through a single outpatient clinic has grown into the Bangladesh Institute of Research and Rehabilitation in Diabetes, Endocrine and Metabolic Disorders (BIRDEM), situated in Dhaka. This organization treated over 71 thousand outpatients in 1998–1999, over 16 thousand of them new attenders.

The impact on clinical practice of rising numbers of people with diabetes has led to the establishment of a National Diagnostic Network as an experimental attempt to make the service run from BIRDEM more accessible to patients by providing quality diagnostic services at a reasonable cost throughout the country. This project combines, amongst other things, the availability of free services to those who need them, paying services in certain centres for those who can afford to pay and the introduction of a health-care package to provide as comprehensive a service as possible. Of great significance in the evolution of non-communicable disease epidemiology is the need that has been felt for the establishment of the Cardiac Center Project.

The key role played by BIRDEM is essential in a poor country where many cannot afford to pay for their health care. BIRDEM is well advanced in the development of the public–private mix of funding that recognizes the need for pragmatic solutions to fund an institute which is, increasingly, expanding its activities and expertise outside the field of diabetes – its initial focus and raison d'être.[28] The future challenges facing low-income countries with growing burdens of non-communicable diseases such as diabetes alongside existing communicable disease, are immense. The BIRDEM model is unique in such countries in combining the established platform of a centralized service in the capital city with an expanding outreach programme aimed at increasing access to specialist care, and in expanding the capacity of the system to deal with increasing numbers of people with diabetes and its complications.

United Kingdom

The National Service Framework (NSF) for diabetes, due to be published in 2001, will pose significant challenges for organizations concerned with delivering primary and secondary care to people with diabetes. These implications need to be seen in the context of changing trends in the delivery of diabetic services in primary care and the more specialist role of secondary care, as well as in relation to the development of Primary Care Groups and Primary Care Trusts (PCG/PCT) in England (and their equivalents elsewhere in the UK) and the future care trusts. These changes will have clinical implications by placing considerable demands on a range of resources, including workload, financial and staffing, in both primary and secondary care.

The implications for diabetes care are likely to range from communication and raising awareness, amongst professionals, changing trends and new diagnostic criteria, through to training needs and the increased resources required throughout the National Health Service (NHS) to deliver an excellent diabetes service. The process of education and raising awareness amongst staff has to be effected in both primary and secondary care and requires time, manpower and financial resources. The NSF may provide the details of the information required to be disseminated within primary and secondary care, and should meet the resources needed to perform this function. The following discussion attempts to consider some of these implications for primary and secondary care.

Implications for Primary Care

Current knowledge and expertise about diabetes care in primary care is patchy. However, a recent meta-analysis of research trials considering care of diabetes in primary care has shown that, given structured care and adequate follow-up arrangements, the standard of care in that sector is as good as the care provided in secondary care diabetes clinics.[29] National surveys of the structural provision of diabetes care in general practice have been carried out and are currently in progress.[30] These suggest that c. 70% of practices hold a specific clinic for people with diabetes, but expertise and resources available for these clinics are, as suggested above, patchy. With or without such clinics, 90% of patient contacts begin and end in primary care. Since the 1990 contract for the management of chronic disease more diabetes has been managed in primary care.[31]

With the increasing prevalence and new criteria it is likely that more people will be tested and be diagnosed with diabetes and IFG. This has major clinical and resource implications for practices and commissioners of services. Currently, patients wishing to join a practice undergo a new patient check that allows for a decision to be made about the risks of developing diabetes and arrangement of further tests if required. Urine analysis has low sensitivity and specificity for detecting diabetes and, in view of the new criteria, it is likely that fasting blood glucose may be performed in high-risk groups. This has implications for the practice in increased nursing time, more appointments and increased pathology costs.

This increased demand would be occurring in the face of ongoing pressures with issues relating to a primary care-led NHS, the National Plan for the NHS, and clinical governance requirements placing considerable strains on primary care to meet targets and improve outcomes for existing people with diabetes. This is likely to be further compounded by the prescribed need to identify people who have diabetes but have not yet been diagnosed and by information contained within the NSF. This will also have resource implications for primary care in terms of communication, structural organization, staffing, numbers of clinics, frequency and number of blood tests, prescribing budgets and others.

It cannot be assumed that the epidemiological trends and changes in criteria have been communicated to all primary care staff and so there is the issue of raising awareness in primary care and any associated training this may require. The process of raising awareness and training has resource implications for PCT and practices. Once awareness is raised this is usually followed by staff being more proactive in identifying people with diabetes. The new diagnostic criteria – leading to an overall increase in the number of people diagnosed with diabetes – will mean more time devoted to diabetes care in the practice, which may in turn have an adverse impact on other general medical services delivered in general practice.

There is a national shortage of general practitioners (GPs) at the present time and this trend is likely to continue, although more doctors are being trained as set out in the NHS Plan but these increases are unlikely to meet the requirements of service expectations. Increased clinical requirements due to increased numbers of people with diabetes will mean the need for longer consultations. To put this into context, an increase of 1 minute of average consultation time equates to an increase of 9.7% in provision of GP time and would correspond to an increase of 3000 GPs to compensate. The increase in the number of people with diabetes being diagnosed earlier means that more staff are required to spend more time caring for people with this condition; therefore, new models of delivering care in diabetes should be sought.

Implications for secondary care

Apart from those stable patients managed in clinics in primary care, most people with diabetes, and those with significant complications of diabetes, are currently managed in secondary care. There are examples of innovative service developments in primary care, e.g. the intermediate care satellite service model in Bradford. This model uses specialist GPs located in the community with complementary teams made up of dieticians, diabetic specialist nurses, practice nurses and podiatrists. Apart from this model, most people with diabetes requiring insulin or who are poorly controlled are referred to the local secondary care diabetes clinic.

Based on current trends of a rising prevalence and earlier diagnosis of diabetes, serious problems for secondary care will develop if resources are not increased or if effective primary prevention is not introduced. On current predictions, the number of diabetologists is insufficient to provide the level of service required and this is before the identification of some of the people with diabetes as yet undiagnosed.

The implications of having greater numbers attending hospital for their diabetes care delivered by highly trained specialists are great. Use of the new diagnostic criteria is likely to mean that more people will be diagnosed earlier than before and will necessitate resource-intensive education, counselling and follow-up. Resources, when translated into people, mean additional diabetologists, dieticians, diabetic specialist nurses, podiatrists and other clinicians involved in diabetes care. It is apparent that either substantial financial, and manpower, resources must be provided for secondary care or a different model for managing diabetes is needed to compensate for increased demand for the service to be met. There is no question that resources will need to be forthcoming for this to happen but alternative models of care will also need to be considered to ease the burden of diabetes on secondary care. These developments will have to be evaluated carefully while ensuring an integration of primary and secondary care diabetes services, better information technologies, and adequate resources to both primary and secondary care and the NHS as a whole.

References

1. American Diabetes Association: the Expert Committee on the Diagnosis and Classification of Diabetes Mellitus. Report of the Expert Committee on the Diagnosis and Classification of Diabetes Mellitus. Diabetes Care 1997; 20:1183–97.

2. World Health Organization. Definition, diagnosis and classification of diabetes mellitus and its complications. Part 1: diagnosis and classification of diabetes mellitus. Diabet Med 1998; 15:539–53.

3. World Health Organization. Diabetes mellitus: report of a WHO study group, Geneva, Switzerland, 1985.

4. Davies M, Kawaguchu Y, Bennet S, et al. A genome-wide search for human Type 1 diabetes susceptibility genes. Nature 1994; 371: 130–6.

5. Leslie R, Pozzilli P. Type I diabetes mascarading as type II diabetes. Diabetes Care 1994; 17:1214–19.

6. Tuomi T, Groop L, Zimmet P, et al. Antibodies to glutamic acid decarboxylase reveal latent autoimmune diabetes mellitus in adults with a non-insulin-dependent onset of the disease. Diabetes 1993; 42: 359–62.

7. Amos A, McCarty DL, Zimmet P. The rising global burden of diabetes and its complications: estimates and projections to the year 2010. Diabet Med 1997; 14: S1–S85.

8. King H, Aubert RE, Herman WH. Global burden of diabetes, 1995–2025. Diabetes Care 1998; 21:1414–31.

9. International Diabetes Federation. Diabetes Atlas 2000. Brussels: International Diabetes Federation; 2000.

10. Williams R. Ascertainment, prevalence, incidence and temporal trends. In: Ekoé J-M, Zimmet P, Williams R, editors. The epidemiology of diabetes. Chichester: Wiley & Sons; 2001.

11. Ruwaard D, Hoogenveen RT, Verkleij H, et al. Forecasting the number of diabetic patients in The Netherlands in 2005. Am J Public Health 1993; 83:989–95.

12. Mokdad A, Ford E, Bowman B, et al. The continuing increase of diabetes in the US. Diabetes Care 2001; 24:412.

13. Mokdad A, Serdula M, Dietz B, et al. The spread of the obesity epidemic in the US. J Am Med Ass 2001; 23: 1278–83.

14. Feltbower R, McKinney P, Bodansky H. Rising incidence of childhood diabetes is seen at all ages and in urban and rural settings in Yorkshire, United Kingdom. Diabetologia 2000; 43:682–4.

15. Schoenle E, Lang-Muritanl M, Gschwend S, et al. Epidemiology of Type 1 diabetes mellitus in Switzerland: steep rise in incidence in under 5 year old children in the past decade. Diabetologia 2001; 44:286–9.

16. Pinhas-Hamiel O, Dolan M, Daniels S, et al. Increased incidence of non-insulin-dependant diabetes mellitus among adolescents. J Paediat 2000; 128:608–15.

17. Kitiwaga T, Owada M, Urakami T,

Yamauchi K. Increased incidence of non-insulin dependant diabetes mellitus among Japanese schoolchildren correlates with an increased intake of animal protein and fat. Clin Paediat 1998; 37: 111–16.

18. American Diabetes Association. Type 2 diabetes in children and adolescents. Paediatrics 2000; 105:671–80.

19. Ehtisham S, Barrett T, Shaw N. Type 2 diabetes in UK children – an emerging problem. Diabet Med 2000; 17:867–71.

20. Unwin N, Alberti KGMM, Bhopal RS, et al. Comparison of the current WHO and new ADA criteria for the diagnosis of diabetes mellitus in three ethnic groups in the UK. Diabet Med 1998; 15:554–7.

21. Davies M, Muehlbayer S, Garrick P, McNally P. Potential impact of a change in the diagnostic criteria for diabetes mellitus on the prevalence of abnormal glucose tolerance in a local community at risk of diabetes: impact of new diagnostic criteria for diabetes mellitus. Diabet Med 1999; 16: 343–6.

22. Kannel WB, McGee DL. Diabetes and glucose tolerance as risk factors for cardiovascular disease: the Framingham study. Diabetes Care 1979; 2: 120–6.

23. Davies M, Raymond N, Day J, et al. Impaired glucose tolerance and fasting hyperglycaemia have different characteristics. Diabet Med 2000; 17: 433–40.

24. Tuomilehto J, Korhonen H, Kartovaara L, et al. Prevalence of diabetes mellitus and impaired glucose tolerance in the middle-aged population of three areas in Finland. Int J Epidem 1991; 20: 1010–17.

25. Aro A. Health services for the diabetic in Finland. In Mann J, Pyorala K, Teuscher A, editors. Diabetes in epidemiological perspective. Edinburgh: Churchill Livingstone; 1983:293–304.

26. Kangas T. The Finndiab Report: health care of people with diabetes in Finland. Stakes National Research and Development Centre for Welfare and Health. Research Reports; 1995.

27. Diabetic Association of Bangladesh (DAB). Diabetic Association of Bangladesh – Annual report 1998–1999. DAB, 1999.

28. Ali L. Public–private mix in Bangladesh: an analysis. Presented at the Annual Conference of the Health Economics Unit, Ministry of Health and Family Welfare, Dhaka, July 1999.

29. Griffin S. Diabetes care in general practice: meta-analysis of randomized control trials. Br Med J 1998; 317:390–5.

30. Pierce M, Agarwal G, Ridout D. The state of two nations: diabetes care in general practice in England and Wales. Presented at the 34th European Diabetes Epidemiology Group, Verona, Italy, 1999.

31. Greenhalgh PM. Shared care for diabetes. a systematic review. London: The Royal College of General Practitioners; occasional paper 1994.

2

Diabetes and obesity: what is the relationship to cardiovascular disease?

Amit Allahabadia and Sudhesh Kumar

Introduction

Type 2 diabetes is set to become one of the great global public health challenges of the early twenty-first century, stretching health-care resources not only of industrialized countries but increasingly also of nations of the developing world. The prevalence of diabetes is increasing rapidly and it is estimated that the number of diabetics worldwide will double by the year 2010. Projections published in 1997 by the International Diabetes Institute indicate there will be more than 230 million people with diabetes by 2010 and the majority of these will have Type 2 diabetes.[1] The most alarming consequence of the rising prevalence of diabetes is its increasing contribution to the overall burden of cardiovascular disease (CVD), by far the commonest cause of death and disability. Excess vascular mortality in diabetes occurs as a consequence of premature onset of atheroma and affects not only the coronary arteries but also the cerebral and peripheral circulation. More than 50% of diabetic patients have evidence of CVD at diagnosis, and CVD is responsible for more than three quarters of all deaths in Type 2 diabetic patients, largely as a result of myocardial infarction and stroke.

The major driving force behind the present epidemic of diabetes is the dramatic worldwide increase in obesity. It is estimated from the third National Health and Nutrition Examination Survey (NHANES III) that the prevalence of obesity in the population of the USA rose to 33% in the period from 1988 to 1991, compared with 25% during the period from 1976 to 1980 (NHANES II),[2] with a similar increase reported in the UK population.[3] Several epidemiological surveys and prospective longitudinal studies have demonstrated that obesity is major risk factor for the development of Type 2 diabetes.[4–6] Whilst obesity is uncommon in Type 1 diabetes mellitus, 75–85% of Type 2 diabetic patients are either overweight or obese. The presence of obesity predisposes affected individu-

15

Table 2.1 Metabolic and cardiovascular risk factors associated with obesity

Insulin resistance
Hyperinsulinaemia
Low high-density lipoprotein cholesterol
High triglyceride concentrations
Increased Apo B concentrations
Small, dense low-density lipoprotein cholesterol
Increased fibrinogen concentrations
Increased plasminogen activator
Increased inhibitor C-reactive protein
Increased C-reactive protein
Increased systolic and diastolic blood pressures
Increased blood viscosity
Increased left ventricular hypertrophy
Premature atherosclerosis (cardiovascular disease and stroke)

als to a variety of other comorbid conditions but, in particular, significantly increases the risk of CVD.[7] During the last two decades, increasing evidence has emerged that obesity is an independent risk factor for CVD. Moreover, it markedly enhances the CVD risk associated with other risk factors such as hypertension and dyslipidaemia, which are associated with Type 2 diabetes in the metabolic syndrome (Table 2.1).[8]

Although both Type 1 and Type 2 diabetes predispose to CVD, the risk appears to be greatest in Type 2 diabetes, which also accounts for the vast majority of cases of diabetes mellitus. In this review the authors focus mainly on Type 2 diabetes, and explore evidence for Type 2 diabetes and obesity as risk factors for CVD. Also examined are the relationships of diabetes and obesity with other coexisting elements of the metabolic syndrome, including insulin resistance, hypertension, dyslipidaemia and thrombotic factors, which are additional risk factors for CVD.

Type 2 diabetes and cardiovascular disease (CVD)

Diabetes as a risk factor for cardiovascular disease (CVD)

Diabetes mellitus has long been recognized as a risk factor for the development of CVD and for excess mortality due to CVD. This observation is derived from strong epidemiological data that show not only an excess of CVD in the diabetic population but also worst outcomes after vascular events in diabetic patients. In the USA, from the early 1970s to the early 1980s, there was a substantial decline in mortality from coronary heart disease in the nondiabetic adult population. During the same period, however, the decrease was considerably less in adults with diabetes.[9] The decline in CVD mortality in the general population of the USA has been attributed to a reduction in cardiovascular risk factors and improvements in the treatment of heart disease; however, the smaller declines in mortality for diabetic subjects indicates that these changes have been less effective for people with diabetes. Several population-based observational studies have confirmed diabetes mellitus as a risk factor for CVD with a two- to fourfold increase in the risk of death from coronary artery disease in diabetic patients compared with their nondiabetic counterparts.[10–15] Most of these studies have also shown that the increased risk of CVD mortality is significantly greater in women than in men,[10,12–14] demonstrating that the cardioprotective effect of female gender is eliminated in diabetes. The magnitude of diabetes as a risk factor for the development of CVD is highlighted clearly by data from Finland, which show that men with diabetes and no history of myocardial infarction have the same likelihood of coronary events as men without diabetes who have previously had such an event.[16] The overall consequence of the excess mortality from CVD is a reduction in life expectancy of at least 5–10 years.

Coronary artery disease is generally more severe in diabetic patients than in nondiabetic patients with CVD and is associated with a poorer outcome.[17–19] Patients develop heart disease at a younger age, have a higher rate of diffuse multivessel disease and are more likely to develop congestive heart failure.[20] Furthermore, outcome following a myocardial infarction tends to be worse with higher rates of cardiac failure and death in the early post-infarction period;[19] similar findings are also evident several years after a coronary event.[21] Data from the Organization to Assess Strategies for Ischemic Syndromes (OASIS) study showed increased mortality in patients with diabetes for several years after a coronary event, most typically from congestive heart failure, despite similar degrees of cardiac dysfunction initially.[21] This suggests that diabetes itself decreases the functional reserve of the heart or it increases the rate of subsequent infarction. Several combined mechanisms are thought to reduce the compensatory ability of the noninfarcted myocardium so that cardiac failure ensues. Postulated mechanisms include pre-existing congestive heart failure caused by diabetic cardiomyopathy, severe coronary artery disease, decreased vasodilatory reserve of epicardial and resistance arteries, and possibly abnormal metabolism of myocardial substrate. Late mortality results from increased reinfarction rates caused by the diffuse nature of the atherosclerotic disease and a hypercoagulable state. Platelet hyperactivity, reduced fibrinolytic capacity, increased concentrations of haemostatic proteins and endothelial dysfunction promote thrombosis at the site of plaque rupture. In addition, autonomic neuropathy predisposes patients to ventricular arrhythmias. The prehospitalization mortality rate from myocardial infarction is also significantly higher in diabetic patients, thereby reducing the opportunity for intervention in an acute event.[22]

The prevalence of CVD is higher in diabetic patients but considerable variations exist in the pattern of CVD in different ethnic groups worldwide. Ethnic groups with a low prevalence of CVD in the nondiabetic population, such as the Japanese, also typically have low rates in diabetics, although with an increased relative risk in diabetic patients.[23] Conversely, ethnic groups with a high prevalence of CVD in the nondiabetic population, such as in the USA and Western Europe, usually have a significantly higher prevalence of CVD in diabetics. There are certain racial groups where the prevalence of diabetes is very high but the risk of developing CVD is relatively low. One such group is the Pima Indians of North America, who have the highest prevalence of diabetes in the world but in whom the rate of death from CVD is less than in the nondiabetic population in the Framingham Study.[24] The most likely reasons for this unexpected finding include genetic factors, low concentrations of low-density lipoproteins (LDL) and total cholesterol, and a low rate of smoking. In contrast, people who originated from the Indian subcontinent and have migrated to industrialized nations have some of the highest rates of CVD in the world.[25]

Hyperglycaemia

Type 2 diabetes is associated with a constellation of risk factors for CVD, most notably dyslipidaemia and hypertension. The question that remains, however, is to what extent, if any, is the association between diabetes and vascular disease independently mediated by hyperglycemia? Hyperglycaemia is well established as a risk factor for small vessel disease in diabetes. Evidence from the Diabetes Complications and Control Trial Research Group showed that the degree of hyperglycaemia and glycaemic control in diabetic patients correlates with the risk and severity of microvascular complications, and that improving hyperglycaemia reduces the risk of development and progression of such complications.[26] There are good theoretical reasons to suggest that hyperglycaemia is also an independent risk factor for the development of large vessel disease and therefore CVD. Improvements in the understanding of the mechanisms by which hyperglycaemia directly causes tissue damage, e.g. through processes such as glyco-oxidation, protein kinase C activation and cellular myoinositol depletion, further implicate it as a factor capable of inducing macrovascular and cardiac damage. The confirmation of hyperglycaemia as a risk factor for CVD is made difficult by the fact that Type 2 diabetes is a progressive condition and, with time a number of confounding variables may become present that also influence CVD risk. Hence, patients with more severe hyperglycaemia are likely to be older, to have had diabetes for longer and may also have renal disease. Observational studies in diabetic populations that have examined hyperglycaemia as a risk factor for CVD have produced conflicting results. In several large studies, no relationship was found between either the duration or the severity of hyperglycaemia and the risk of CVD,[27–29] whereas in others only a modest effect was detected.[30]

It was not until the publication of the United Kingdom Prospective Diabetes Study (UKPDS) in 1998 that hyperglycaemia and the improvement of glycaemic control was shown, for the first time, to be associated with the risk of CVD.[31,32] This study reported the effects of intensive treatment of hyperglycaemia in 3867 newly diagnosed Type 2 diabetic patients over a 10-year period. Subjects were randomized to a regimen of conventional or intensive treatment: patients in the conventional group were treated initially with diet alone, although drugs were allowed if control deteriorated beyond a certain point; the intensively treated group were managed with oral hypoglycaemic agents or insulin. Over the period of the study there was 0.9% difference in glycated haemoglobin between the two groups studied, 7.9% in the conventional group and 7.0% in the intensive one. This difference in control was associated with significant benefits in microvascular disease with a 25% reduction in the development of microvascular end-points ($p < 0.01$) and a 12% reduction in any diabetes-related complication ($p < 0.029$). The incidence of cardiovascular disease was not significantly reduced, although a reduction of 16% in the intensively treated group compared with the conventional group was almost significant ($p = 0.052$). However, the subgroup of patients treated intensively with metformin had a 39% reduction in the incidence of myocardial infarction compared with the conventional group and those in the intensively treated group who received insulin or a sulphonylurea. There is less data for Type 1 diabetes, but here too it appears likely that the level of blood glucose is a cardiovascular risk factor.[33]

Although hyperglycaemia is now a recognized risk factor for coronary artery disease, it was not clear until recently whether elevated fasting glucose or postprandial hyperglycaemia is more important as a determinant of cardiovascular risk. Evidence from several recent large epidemiological studies suggest that postprandial hyperglycaemia (post-meal hyperglycaemic peaks), measured by the 2 hour glucose concentration of an oral glucose tolerance test, may be more strongly related to CVD morbidity and mortality than the fasting blood glucose concentration.[34–36]

It is clear from the UKPDS that long-term glycaemic control influences the risk of CVD and the mortality from it. Strong evidence also exists from the Diabetes and Insulin–Glucose Infusion in Acute Myocardial Infarction (DIGAMI) study that acute intensive control of hyperglycaemia at the time of and after a myocardial infarction influences subsequent survival.[37] In this trial, patients were randomized to an intensive insulin therapy group treated with an insulin–glucose infusion for at least 24 hours followed by an intensive insulin treatment regimen at discharge or to a control group managed with conventional therapy. The mortality rate at a 3-year follow-up was 33% in the intensively treated group compared with 44% in the conventional group (p = 0.011). Several mechanisms have been postulated for the improvement in mortality, including direct effects of large amounts of insulin on the reduction of metabolic risk factors (such as impaired platelet function, lipoproteins abnormalities, prothrombotic factors) and the removal of potential cardiotoxic effects of sulphonylureas and metformin. It is likely, therefore, that the benefits seen in the DIGAMI study are not due to a glucose effect.

Blood glucose concentrations at the time of a myocardial infarction clearly influence subsequent CVD morbidity and mortality in diabetic patients but may also be important in nondiabetic patients. A recent meta-analysis showed that patients without diabetes who had glucose concentrations ≥ 6.1–8.0mmol/l had a 3.9-fold higher risk of death than patients without diabetes who had lower glucose concentrations.[38] Therefore, a potential intervention clearly exists in such patients to lower blood glucose concentrations in order to improve survival post-myocardial infarction. Twenty years before the DIGAMI study, de Micheli et al.[39] proposed the use of insulin infusions in patients without diabetes, following experiments in dogs that demonstrated a cardioprotective effect.[39] Although clinical trials have since been conducted, the results have been inconclusive, most likely due to small numbers of patients and the different protocols used in these studies. Meta-analysis of such studies suggests that this treatment may be effective but larger prospective studies are clearly required to determine any benefit.[40]

Obesity and cardiovascular disease (CVD)

Definition of obesity and risk of morbidity

Most clinicians are aware that patients with Type 2 diabetes are usually overweight or obese, but what is obesity and how is it defined? Obesity is, in simple terms, an excess storage of body fat. It develops from an excess of energy intake compared with energy expenditure. In adult men of average weight, fat comprises 15–20% of the total body weight, while in women this proportion is greater at c. 25–30%. The precise definition of obesity, or being overweight, remains somewhat arbitrary and controversial for a number of reasons. First, the distribution of weight within a given population forms a continuous curve rather than division into discrete populations of obese and non-obese individuals.[41] Second, because differences in weight between individuals relate not only to variations in body fat but also frame size and muscle bulk, many observers dispute the use of absolute weight or measures based upon height and weight [such as the body mass index (BMI)] to differentiate between normal and overweight individuals. Despite this latter argument, epidemiological evidence from large populations has demonstrated that there is an excellent correlation between BMI [defined as weight in kilograms divided by height in metres squared (kg/m^2)] and the percentage of body fat in large populations.[42,43] In clinical practice, individuals or populations are not classified on the basis of body fat percentage but on the basis of their BMI. The measurement of BMI also reflects the risk of mortality with variation in weight and, as a result, in 1995 the World Health Organization (WHO) proposed cut-off points for the classification of obesity according to mortality risk (Table 2.2).

During the last 50 years it has become apparent that different body morphology, or types of fat distribution, are independently related to the health risks associated with obesity. Substantial evidence now indicates that accumulation of fat in a central or upper body distribution predicts comorbidities and mortality from obesity.[44] Unfortunately, a BMI-based definition fails to take body fat distribution into account. Fat accumulation in the upper body, which has variously been described as central, truncal or visceral obesity, may be measured by an increased waist circumference or more popularly, a waist-to-hip circumference ratio. The relationship between the ratio of the waist-to-hip circumference and CVD end-points, including myocardial infarction, angina pectoris, stroke and death, have been shown to be stronger than for any other anthropometric variable in a number of studies.[44,45]

WHO criteria that define overweight and obesity in terms of comorbidities are not necessarily appropriate for Asian populations.[46] A working party with representation from WHO, the International Society for the Study of Obesity and the International Obesity Task Force has recently recommended new criteria for defining obesity in the Asian population. In Asians a BMI range of $23–24.9 kg/m^2$ has an equivalent risk of Type 2 diabetes, hypertension and dyslipidaemia as a BMI of $25–29.9 kg/m^2$ in Europeans.

Table 2.2 Classification of overweight and obesity in adults according to body mass index (BMI)*

BMI (kg/m^2)	WHO Classification	Popular description
< 18.5	Underweight	Thin
18.5–24.9	–	Healthy or normal
25.0–29.9	Grade 1 overweight	Overweight
30.0–39.9	Grade 2 overweight	Obesity
⩾ 40.0	Grade 3 overweight	Morbid obesity

*Adapted from WHO

Generalized obesity and cardiovascular risk

Until recently, the relationship between obesity and coronary heart disease (CHD) was viewed as indirect, mediated through other risk factors related to both obesity and CHD risk, including hypertension, dyslipidaemia and impaired glucose tolerance or noninsulin-dependent diabetes mellitus. Insulin resistance and accompanying hyperinsulinaemia are usually associated with these risk factors. A number of cross-sectional and prospective studies have suggested that excessive body fat is closely associated with, and independently predicts, premature cardiovascular mortality and morbidity in overweight individuals. These studies have examined the impact of excess weight in adult life as well in childhood and adolescence. Evidence for a relationship between obesity and cardiovascular disease was first suggested by epidemiological studies. In the Framingham Heart Study,[47] the relationship between obesity and cardiovascular disease was examined after a follow-up period of 26 years.[47] Excess weight (Metropolitan Relative Weight) was found to be an independent predictor for coronary disease, coronary death and congestive heart failure in men after adjusting for other recognized risk factors. Relative weight in women was also positively and independently associated with coronary disease, stroke, congestive failure, and coronary and cardiovascular death. This study also showed that weight gain after the young adult years conveyed an increased risk of CVD in both sexes that could not be attributed either to the initial weight or the levels of the risk factors that may have resulted from weight gain. The prospective Nurses Health Study, which investigated more than 115,000 women in the USA during a follow-up period of 16 years, found that death rates from cardiovascular disease among obese individuals (BMI $\geq$ 29kg/m^2) were increased fourfold compared with the leanest women.[48]

There is also increasing evidence that overweight children and adolescents are at increased risk of premature death and morbidity from all causes, in particular from cardiovascular disease. Long-term follow-up from the Harvard Growth Study of 1922–1935, revealed that subjects who were overweight in adolescence had an associated increased risk of mortality from all causes and disease-specific mortality among men but not among women.[49] The relative risks among men were 1.8 for mortality from all causes and 2.3 for mortality from CHD. The risk of morbidity from CHD and atherosclerosis was, however, increased among men and women who had been overweight in adolescence. Excessive weight in adolescence was a more powerful predictor of these risks than excessive weight in adulthood. In the UK, a 57 year follow-up of 2990 subjects [Carnegie Survey of Family Diet and Health in pre-war Britain (1937–1939)] revealed that childhood BMI above the 75th centile was associated with a relative risk of 2 for ischaemic heart disease compared with a BMI between the 25th and 49th centiles.[50] As in the study in the

USA, there was also an increase in the all-cause mortality. An excess risk of cardiovascular disease with increased BMI has recently been shown to be greatest in young adulthood and appears to decline with increasing age in a cohort of more than 360,000 subjects[51]

The impact of weight gain on cardiovascular risk has been demonstrated unequivocally in the Framingham Heart and the Nurses Health Studies. In the Framingham Heart Study, weight gain after young adulthood increased cardiovascular risk in men and women such that this could not be attributed to the initial weight or to the risk factors that may have occurred due to weight gain. The Nurses Health Study showed that relative risk of cardiovascular morbidity and mortality increases with increasing BMI at age 18.[48] Furthermore, each kilogram of weight gain from the age of 18 years was associated with a 3.1% higher relative risk of cardiovascular disease.[52]

In a more recent study, Ashton et al.[53] investigated the relationship between BMI and several established risk factors for coronary heart disease in a cross-sectional survey of more than 14,000 apparently healthy women. They found that as BMI increased from < 20 to > 30, blood pressure also increased significantly, as did concentrations of total cholesterol, LDL cholesterol, apolipoprotein B, fasting triglycerides and fasting blood glucose, while high-density lipoprotein (HDL) cholesterol and apolipoprotein A1 decreased. Using a modified version of the Framingham Heart Study's algorithm for predicting the risk of CHD, the investigators showed that the estimated 10-year risk of CHD also increased significantly in a dose-responsive fashion as BMI increased from < 20 to > 30. The data in this study are important in that they provide mechanistic support for the direct, linear association between BMI and CVD risk seen in prospective cohort studies in Western populations. Furthermore, they suggest that the adverse metabolic consequences of adiposity may exist on a continuum and that even small increases in body weight in the lower to middle range of the BMI distribution (< 25) may translate into important increases in the long-term risk of CHD.

Fat distribution as a determinant of cardiovascular risk

BMI is the most commonly used clinical measure of obesity but it fails to take body fat distribution into account. Body fat distribution was first postulated as a factor for health risk more than 40 years ago.[54] Several longitudinal studies have since examined the distribution of body fat for association with cardiovascular disease.[44,45] These prospective studies have shown that central (truncal) body fat deposition is associated with increased cardiovascular morbidity and mortality, independent of generalized obesity (defined by BMI).[44] Moreover, central obesity is a better predictor of cardiovascular disease and death than the degree of obesity. The waist-to-hip circumference ratio was used as a measure of central obesity and was found to be associated with occurrence of stroke, ischaemic heart disease and death from all causes in men,[45] and with a 12-year incidence of myocardial infarction, angina, stroke and death in women.[44]

Although regional obesity is highly predictive of cardiovascular disease and poor outcome, the reasons for this relationship are still unclear. It is has been hypothesized that intraperitoneal adipose tissue is predominantly responsible for the development of insulin resistance because of the higher lipolytic activity (observed within in vitro studies) and because of direct drainage to the liver through the portal circulation as described above.[55]

Left ventricular hypertrophy (LVH) and congestive heart failure

Changes in cardiac structure and function are common in obese subjects, even in the absence of hypertension and underlying organic heart disease. Obesity is associated with increased total blood volume, creating a high cardiac output state that may cause ventricular dilatation and, ultimately, eccentric hypertrophy of the left ventricle (LV).[56] Eccentric LVH produces diastolic dysfunction; systolic dysfunction may ensue due to excessive wall stress if wall thickening fails to keep pace with dilatation. This disorder is often referred to as obesity cardiomyopathy. The presence of hypertension in obese individuals places a dual burden on the LV, facilitating and exacerbating the development of left ventricular dilatation and hypertrophy in concentric and eccentric patterns.[56-58] Congestive heart failure and sudden death are common sequelae of changes in left ventricular structure and function in obese subjects with and without hypertension. Heart failure may be attributable to LV diastolic dysfunction or to combined LV diastolic and systolic dysfunction. The propensity for sudden death is also likely due to these changes within the LV. In a study of 22 patients with severe obesity at post mortem, dilated cardiomyopathy was most frequently associated with sudden death.[59] Dilated cardiomopathy is likely, therefore, to be the most common cause of sudden death in patients with severe obesity. This is presumably due to the occurrence of complex ventricular arrhythmias. The reasons for arrhythmia development are unknown but may relate to a prolonged Q–T interval, which occurs in up to one third of obese subjects and which may, therefore, predispose to such arrhythmias.[60] Furthermore, post mortem and echocardiographic findings in obese subjects reveal fatty infiltration of the conduction system and left atrial enlargement that may also lead to arrhythmias.

Right ventricular dysfunction

Structural and functional changes are not confined to the left side of the heart but also occur in the right heart in obesity. There are thought to be two major mechanisms that underlie right ventricular dysfunction. First, the obstructive sleep apnoea and/or the obesity hypoventilation syndrome occurs in 5% of morbidly obese individuals,[56] causing pulmonary hypertension and right ventricular hypertrophy, dilatation, progressive dysfunction and, finally, right ventricular failure. Right ventricular dysfunction can also occur as a consequence of left ventricular dysfunction and the heart failure that develops is often biventricular.

How does obesity cause cardiovascular disease (CVD)?

Obesity significantly increases the risk of development of CVD; there appears to be a continuous relationship between BMI and the risk of CVD even at moderate BMI levels. Evidence from a number of cross-sectional and longitudinal studies, described above, supports the role of obesity as a major independent risk factor for the development of CVD. Moreover, obesity is strongly associated with and predisposes to a number of other coexisting conditions, including Type 2 diabetes, insulin resistance, hypertension and dyslipidaemia, which further contribute, independently, to the development of CVD. The relationships of obesity with these conditions are discussed below.

Obesity and Type 2 diabetes

The association of central obesity and a clustering of cardiovascular risk factors, including diabetes and hypertension, was noted more than 40 years ago by Vague.[54] Since then a number of epidemiological studies have demonstrated a link between obesity and Type 2 diabetes in high-risk populations[61,62] and white Caucasian patients.[63] The risk of Type 2 diabetes has been shown to rise markedly with increasing degrees of obesity.[4,5,64,65] A large body of evidence exists for a direct and continuous relationship between BMI (kg/m^2) and the risk of developing Type 2 diabetes.[66-68] In the Nurses Health Study, the risk of developing diabetes increased fivefold in women with a BMI of $25kg/m^2$ compared with those whose BMI was $22kg/m^2$.[67] This risk increased to 28-fold for those with a BMI of 30 and 93-fold for those with a BMI > $35kg/m^2$ (Figure 2.1). Similar but smaller risks for equivalent BMI have also been reported in men.[69] Moreover, the distribution of excess fat is an important determinant for developing Type 2 diabetes, with central obesity conferring the greatest magnitude of risk as measured by a high waist-to-hip circumference ratio[45] and waist circumference.[70] In addition to the amount of obesity, the duration of obesity is important and has been shown to be directly related to the risk of diabetes.[71]

Obesity is thought to predispose to Type 2 diabetes through the development of insulin resistance, discussed below.

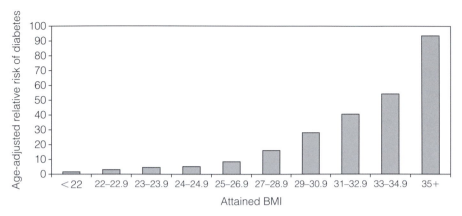

Figure 2.1

Attained body mass index (BMI) and relative risk for noninsulin-dependent diabetes mellitus in women in the USA, between the ages of 30 and 55, in 1976 and followed for 14 years (from the Nurses Health Study[48]).

Obesity and insulin resistance

Insulin resistance is defined as the resistance of body tissues to the bio-logical effects of insulin, reflected in a reduction in the ability of insulin to regulate carbohydrate and lipid metabolism. Insulin resistance is a known feature of obesity and its incidence rises with increasing BMI.[72,73] In addition to generalized obesity, body fat distribution influences insulin resistance. Central obesity is independently associated with insulin resis-tance and the degree of central obesity is directly related to the degree of insulin resistance. Central obesity also reflects accumulation of intra-abdominal visceral fat in the omental and paraintestinal regions. Individ-uals with central obesity are at high risk for hyperinsulinaemia, insulin resistance and Type 2 diabetes.[73–76] Experiments by Bonadonna et al.,[77] using the euglycaemic hyperinsulinaemic clamp technique, revealed that obese individuals have both impaired sensitivity and decreased respon-siveness to insulin compared with their lean counterparts. Furthermore, using a hyperglycaemic clamp, they found that insulin secretion was twice as great in obese subjects as in lean controls but that the insulin did not normalize glucose disposal.

The association between obesity, insulin resistance and Type 2 dia-betes is incompletely understood and several hypotheses have been proposed. One possibility is that obesity mediates its effects on insulin action, plasma insulin concentrations and glucose metabolism by changes in the concentrations of non-esterified fatty acids (NEFA) that exert effects on insulin action at different levels (Figure 2.2). Different body depots of adipose tissue differ in their fatty acid turnover (the

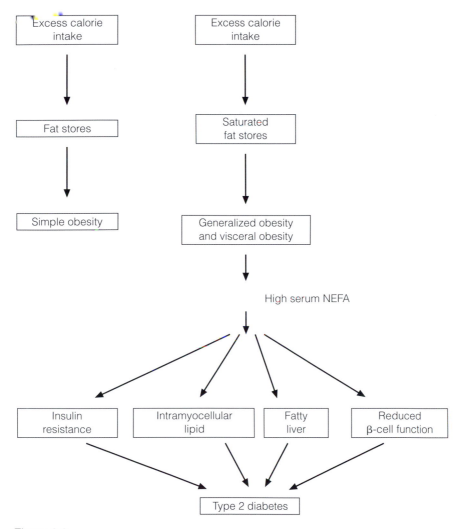

Figure 2.2

Obesity associated insulin resistance and Type 2 diabetes. NEFA, Non-esterified fatty acids.

lipolysis/lipogenesis cycle), and intra-abdominal fat is metabolically active and is associated with increased rates of lipolysis.[78] Therefore, elevated rates of lipolysis in centrally obese individuals lead to increased delivery of NEFA from adipose tissue to skeletal muscle and to the liver via the portal venous circulation. The increased delivery of NEFA to the liver causes hypertriglyceridaemia and reduced hepatic extraction of insulin, leading to hyperinsulinaemia.[79] There is also data that suggests that NEFA independently stimulates glucose production in the liver.[80] High circulating levels of NEFA may also cause insulin resistance by interfering with the insulin-mediated glucose uptake and utilization of glucose in skeletal muscle, resulting in compensatory hyperinsulinaemia (glucose fatty acid cycle).[81]

A second possibility is that cytokines and proteins secreted by adipose tissue may contribute to insulin resistance. Studies in genetically obese animals suggest that increased release of the cytocrine tumour necrosis factor alpha (TNF-α) from adipocytes may play a major role in the impairment of insulin action[82,84] In these studies, administration of anti-TNF-α antibody led to marked improvement in glucose utilization in obese rats,[82] and obese mice genetically lacking TNF-α were found to have more normal insulin sensitivity.[85] More recently, the discovery of resistin, a novel 750 residue protein, suggests that this may be important in the relationship between obesity and diabetes.[86] Resistin is secreted by adipose tissue and levels rise after feeding, and appear to reduce during a period of fasting. Experiments carried out in obese mice show that resistin can induce insulin resistance and glucose intolerance; blocking resistin action by specific antibodies appears to improve insulin resistance and glucose intolerance.[86]

Increasing evidence suggests that insulin resistance, with its associated marker hyperinsulinaemia, is itself a risk factor for CVD,[87] independent of hypertension, atherogenic dyslipidaemia and Type 2 diabetes that coexist in its presence.[88,89] A number of epidemiological studies have previously shown a strong association between raised fasting insulin levels and mortality from CVD in nondiabetic individuals.[90,91] The results of the recent prospective Quebec Heart Study demonstrated the independent effect of hyperinsulinaemia in conferring CVD risk to nondiabetic men.[76] In addition it confirmed association of hyperinsulinaemia with other risk factors for CVD. In individuals without diabetes, the degree of insulin resistance was related to HDL cholesterol (HDL-C) levels, blood pressure and fasting insulin levels. When patients with the highest quintiles of fasting insulin levels compared to those with the lowest quintiles, HDL-C was 12mg/dl lower, blood pressure was 9mmHg higher and triglyceride levels were doubled. After adjusting for these factors, LDL cholesterol (LDL-C) and glucose levels, the most insulin-resistant group demonstrated a 2.5-fold increase in their risk of vascular events.

In addition to association with established risk factors such as dyslipidaemia and hypertension, evidence is emerging of a relationship between obesity and insulin resistance with the presence of inflammation and prothrombotic factors. C-reactive protein (CRP) levels are strongly associated with insulin levels and obesity, although the direction of causality is unclear.[92] CRP is strongly associated with the development of CVD, with a CRP level > 4mg/l associated with a four- to seven-fold increase in risk.[93,94] CRP is also a risk factor for the development of diabetes,[95] with the top quintile of the population demonstrating a 2.5-fold increased risk. Inflammatory factors may, therefore, form part of the association between obesity, diabetes and coronary artery disease.

Increased concentrations of plasminogen activator inhibitor (PAI) have been reported in obese individuals, particularly in those with central obesity.[96] PAI-1 complexes with a tissue-type plasminogen activator, so eliminating its fibrinolytic activity.[97-100] The increased concentrations of PAI-1 are related to hyperinsulinaemia associated with obesity and especially central obesity.[76,101-103] A relative imbalance of the fibrinolytic factors may be associated with early coronary heart disease. Increased concentrations of PAI-1 have been associated with an increased risk of thrombosis in animal and clinical studies.[97-100] Imbalance of fibrinolytic proteins can also have pathogenic consequences within the vascular wall. In vascular tissue, plasmin activates matrix metalloproteases that are crucial in remodelling after vascular injury through degradation of collagen and other glycoproteins that accumulate in plaques.

Obesity and hypertension

One of the most profound effects of obesity on cardiovascular health and disease is hypertension. Epidemiological studies indicate that obesity is a strong independent risk factor for hypertension,[104,105] with a prevalence of hypertension estimated to be 50–300% higher in obese subjects than in normal weight persons.[106] Weight gain has also been shown to be related to increased blood pressure in longitudinal studies.[107] In addition to generalized obesity, body fat distribution appears to be an important determinant of hypertension and again is a more powerful predictor than overall obesity.[108]

The precise mechanisms of hypertension related to obesity are not fully understood. Several hypotheses have been proposed. These include hypervolaemia causing increased cardiac output with failure of reduction in systemic vascular resistance,[109] stimulation of the renin–angiotensin–aldosterone system[110] and increased salt intake due to increased calorie intake.[111] In addition to these mechanisms, it is likely that insulin resistance has significant role in the development of hypertension in obese subjects as hypertension is a major component of the metabolic syndrome. Several mechanisms have been postulated by which insulin resistance and hyperinsulinaemia lead to elevation of blood pressure. One such theory is that increases in plasma insulin concentration stimulate sodium reabsorption by the distal nephron of the kidney. DeFronzo et al.[112] demonstrated that insulin plays a major role in the regulation of renal sodium metabolism and in regulating whole-body sodium homeostasis. It is, therefore, not surprising that obese individuals and those with Type 2 diabetes exhibit impaired excretion of a sodium load. The relationship between insulin resistance and hypertension is not limited to effects on sodium metabolism. Individuals with insulin resistance, especially those who are obese, tend to have activation of the sympathetic nervous system, correlating with elevation of both systolic and diastolic blood pressure.[113] Moreover, hyperinsulinaemia itself stimulates sympathetic nervous system activity via direct action on the central nervous system[114] Hyperinsulinaemia therefore promotes hypertension by dual-role mechanisms of promotion of sodium retention and stimulation of the sympathetic nervous system.

Although the mechanisms linking obesity to hypertension require further investigation, intervention studies have clearly and consistently shown the benefits of weight loss in lowering blood pressure.[109] Weight reduction appears to be the most effective non-pharmacological strategy in the control of blood pressure, with the reduction in blood pressure related to the amount of weight lost. In addition, a number of interventional trials in hypertension have been conducted that have examined effects of lowering blood pressure on CVD risk in diabetic patients. The Hypertension Optimal Treatment (HOT) Study, which examined the benefit of aggressive lowering of blood pressure from 90 to 80mmHg using the calcium antagonist felodipine, found that diabetics who were treated to achieve a diastolic pressure of 80mmHg had fewer CVD events and a lower mortality than those with a diastolic pressure of 90mmHg.[115] In the UKPDS, tight control of blood pressure using either captopril or atenolol (mean 144/82mmHg) achieved a 21% reduction in the incidence of myocardial infarction, although this did not reach statistical significance.[31,32] However, the incidence of stroke and microvascular complications were significantly reduced by 44 and 37%, respectively. A combination of weight reduction and pharmacotherapy are, therefore, likely to be successful strategies in reducing CVD risk in hypertensive obese diabetic patients.

Obesity and dyslipidaemia

Several studies have shown that obesity, insulin resistance and Type 2 diabetes are often associated with lipoprotein abnormalities.[116] Increased levels of triglycerides, low plasma levels of HDL-C and qualitative changes in LDL particles (defined as small dense LDL) are often found in obese individuals. Although qualitative changes occur in LDL particles, elevation of LDL-C has not uniformly been described and total cholesterol levels are similar to those in nondiabetic individuals. Kinetic studies have shown that production of very low-density lipoproteins (VLDL) is increased in obese subjects. This increased VLDL production may relate to increased turnover of NEFA in obesity, which stimulates the liver to synthesize more TG-enriched VLDL. Some obese subjects respond to increased VLDL production by increasing their capacity for clearance of VLDL but in others hypertriglyceridaemia may result. Increased concentrations of circulating VLDL particles lead to an increased exchange of VLDL triglycerides for cholesterol esters derived from HDL and LDL. This exchange results in reduced HDL-C concentrations and the formation of atherogenic small, dense cholesterol-depleted LDL. Such qualitative abnormalities in LDL particles is a major contributing factor from the altered lipoprotein profile that leads to increased atherogenic risk in obesity. In patients who have coexisting metabolic abnormalities that affect LDL metabolism, raised concentrations of LDL-C may occur in addition to the qualitative changes.

Lipoprotein abnormalities in obesity vary according to gender, age and race. Changes in HDL-C levels are more pronounced in women than in men. The association between obesity and LDL-C is more complex. LDL-C concentrations increase with BMI in men, but such increases are not as pronounced in women, the elderly and some ethnic groups. Increasing BMI is associated with small, atherogenic LDL. Furthermore, central obesity in women is associated with elevated LDL-C concentrations.

The Multiple Risk Factor Intervention Trial (MRFIT) demonstrated a curvilinear relationship between the total cholesterol value and CHD mortality in diabetic men that was parallel to, but with a fourfold greater risk than, that in men without diabetes.[104] The impact, therefore, of cholesterol on CVD risk in diabetic men is considerably greater than in the nondiabetic population. Many observational and prospective studies have also shown that triglyceride and HDL-C have significantly greater predictive powers for CVD in diabetic subjects than do the total cholesterol or LDL-C values.[117–118]

Benefits of moderate weight loss

There is a strong link between obesity and the development of CVD, as well the presence of other cardiovascular risk factors such as diabetes, hypertension and dyslipidaemia, but does weight loss lead to a reduction in CVD risk? There are no prospective studies that address this important question but several observational studies suggest that even a modest 5–10% weight loss may be associated with significant benefits (Table 2.3). One retrospective UK study in obese patients with Type 2 diabetes or glucose intolerance revealed that an average weight loss of 1kg was associated with an increased survival of 3–4 months.[119] Extrapolating from this, the authors estimated that a weight loss of only 10kg would restore c. 35% of the life expectancy in obese Type 2 diabetics to reach the figure in the healthy population. The increased life expectancy following moderate weight loss observed in this study has been confirmed in several other studies. The beneficial effects of weight loss are likely to be due to the direct effects of reduction in obesity and improvement of other cardiovascular risk factors. Weight reduction leads to measurable

Table 2.3 Benefits of 10kg weight loss

Diabetes	30–50% reduction in fasting blood glucose
	15% reduction in HbA1c
Lipids	10% reduction in total cholesterol
	15% reduction in low-density lipoprotein cholesterol
	30% reduction in triglycerides
	8% increase in high-density lipoprotein cholesterol
Angina	33% increase in exercise tolerance
	90% reduction in symptoms
Mortality	20–25% reduction in total mortality
	30–40% fall in diabetes-related deaths
Blood pressure	10 mmHg reduction in systolic pressure
	20mmHg reduction in diastolic pressure

Adapted from Wilding and Williams.[122]

changes in intravascular blood volume, cardiac preload and afterload pressures, adrenergic activity and insulin resistance. Improvements in glycaemic control have been reported following weight loss[120,121] and this, in turn, would be expected to reduce the risk of macrovascular complications, including CVD. Moderate weight loss has also been shown to have beneficial effects on the established cardiovascular risk factors of hypertension and dyslipidaemia. The effects of moderate weight loss have been extensively reviewed elsewhere and are summarized in Table 2.3.[122] Studies that have demonstrated the potential cardiovascular benefits of weight loss further emphasize the role of obesity in the pathogenesis of cardiovascular disease.

Summary and conclusions

The relationship between obesity, diabetes and CVD is well established. Until the last few years, the significantly increased risk of CVD with obesity and Type 2 diabetes was thought to be mediated through other coexisting risk factors such as hypertension and dyslipidaemia. During the last decade, a number of studies have determined that obesity and hyperglycaemia are independent risk factors that should actively be treated to lessen the burden of CVD morbidity and mortality. In particular, the importance of treating obesity is gaining increasing recognition, as the effects on all of the other coexisting risk factors including hyperglycaemia are profound. In the future a much greater emphasis is needed for treating obesity in diabetic patients.

References

1. Zimmet PZ, McCarty DJ, de Courten MP. The global epidemiology of non-insulin-dependent diabetes mellitus and the metabolic syndrome. J Diabetes Complicat 1997; 11:60–8.

2. Kuczmarski RJ, Flegal KM, Campbell SM, Johnson CL. Increasing prevalence of overweight among US adults. The National Health and Nutrition Examination Surveys, 1960 to 1991. J Am Med Ass 1994; 272: 205–11.

3. Surveys OoPCa. Health Survey for England; London; HMSO: 1991.

4. Lew EA, Garfinkel L. Variations in mortality by weight among 750,000 men and women. J Chronic Dis 1979; 32:563–76.

5. Larsson B, Bjorntorp P, Tibblin G. The health consequences of moderate obesity. Int J Obes 1981; 5:97–116.

6. Colditz GA, Willett WC, Rotnitzky A, Manson JE. Weight gain as a risk factor for clinical diabetes mellitus in women. Ann Intern Med 1995; 122:481–6.

7. Calle EE, Thun MJ, Petrelli JM, et al. Body-mass index and mortality in a prospective cohort of U.S. adults. New Engl J Med 1999; 341: 1097–105.

8. Reaven GM. Banting lecture 1988. Role of insulin resistance in human disease. Diabetes 1988; 37:1595–607.

9. Gu K, Cowie CC, Harris MI. Diabetes and decline in heart disease mortality in US adults. J Am Med Ass 1999; 281:1291–7.

10. Kannel WB, McGee DL. Diabetes and cardiovascular risk factors: the Framingham study. Circulation 1979; 59:8–13.

11. Jarrett RJ, Shipley MJ. Mortality and associated risk factors in diabetics. Acta Endocr (Suppl) 1985; 272:21–6.

12. Pan WH, Cedres LB, Liu K, et al. Relationship of clinical diabetes and asymptomatic hyperglycemia to risk of coronary heart disease mortality in men and women. Am J Epidemiol 1986; 123:504–16.

13. Barrett-Connor E, Wingard DL. Sex differential in ischemic heart disease mortality in diabetics: a prospective population-based study. Am J Epidemiol 1983; 118: 489–96.

14. Pyorala K, Laakso M, Uusitupa M. Diabetes and atherosclerosis: an epidemiologic view. Diabetes Metab Rev 1987; 3:463–524.

15. Manson JE, Colditz GA, Stampfer MJ, et al. A prospective study of maturity-onset diabetes mellitus and risk of coronary heart disease and stroke in women. Archs Intern Med 1991; 151:1141–7.

16. Haffner SM, Lehto S, Ronnemaa T, et al. Mortality from coronary heart disease in subjects with type 2 diabetes and in nondiabetic subjects with and without prior myocardial infarction. New Engl J Med 1998; 339:229–34.

17. Smith JW, Marcus FI, Serokman R. Prognosis of patients with diabetes mellitus after acute myocardial infarction. Am J Cardiol 1984; 54:718–21.

18. Stone PH, Muller JE, Hartwell T, et al. The effect of diabetes mellitus on prognosis and serial left ventricular function after acute myocardial infarction: contribution of both coronary disease and diastolic left ventricular dysfunction to the adverse prognosis. The MILIS Study Group. J Am Coll Cardiol 1989; 14:49–57.

19. Singer DE, Moulton AW, Nathan DM. Diabetic myocardial infarc-

tion. Interaction of diabetes with other preinfarction risk factors. Diabetes 1989; 38:350–7.

20. Aronson D, Rayfield EJ, Chesebro JH. Mechanisms determining course and outcome of diabetic patients who have had acute myocardial infarction. Ann Intern Med 1997; 126:296–306.

21. Organization to Assess Strategies for Ischemic Syndromes (OASIS) Investigators. Comparison of the effects of two doses of recombinant hirudin compared with heparin in patients with acute myocardial ischemia without ST elevation: a pilot study. Circulation 1997; 96:769–77.

22. Miettinen H, Lehto S, Salomaa V, et al. Impact of diabetes on mortality after the first myocardial infarction. The FINMONICA Myocardial Infarction Register Study Group. Diabetes Care 1998; 21:69–75.

23. Sasaki A, Horiuchi N, Hasegawa K, Uehara M. Mortality and causes of death in type 2 diabetic patients. A long-term follow-up study in Osaka District, Japan. Diabetes Res Clin Pract 1989; 7: 33–40.

24. Nelson RG, Sievers ML, Knowler WC, et al. Low incidence of fatal coronary heart disease in Pima Indians despite high prevalence of non-insulin-dependent diabetes. Circulation 1990;81: 987–95.

25. McKeigue PM, Miller GJ, Marmot MG. Coronary heart disease in south Asians overseas: a review. J Clin Epidemiol 1989; 42: 597–609.

26. The Diabetes Control and Complications Trial Research Group. The effect of intensive treatment of diabetes on the development and progression of long-term complications in insulin-dependent diabetes mellitus. New Engl

J Med 1993; 329:977–86.

27. West KM, Ahuja MM, Bennett PH, et al. The role of circulating glucose and triglyceride concentrations and their interactions with other 'risk factors' as determinants of arterial disease in nine diabetic population samples from the WHO multinational study. Diabetes Care 1983; 6:361–9.

28. Morrish NJ, Stevens LK, Head J, et al. A prospective study of mortality among middle-aged diabetic patients (the London Cohort of the WHO Multinational Study of Vascular Disease in Diabetics) I: Causes and death rates. Diabetologia 1990; 33:538–41.

29. Wilson PW, Cupples LA, Kannel WB . Is hyperglycemia associated with cardiovascular disease? The Framingham Study. Am Heart J 1991; 121:586–90.

30. Klein R. Hyperglycemia and microvascular and macrovascular disease in diabetes. Diabetes Care 1995; 18:258–68.

31. UK Prospective Diabetes Study (UKPDS) Group. Intensive blood-glucose control with sulphonylureas or insulin compared with conventional treatment and risk of complications in patients with type 2 diabetes (UKPDS 33). Lancet 1998; 352:837–53.

32. Turner RC, Millns H, Neil HA, et al. Risk factors for coronary artery disease in non-insulin dependent diabetes mellitus: United Kingdom Prospective Diabetes Study (UKPDS: 23). Br Med J 1998; 316:823–8.

33. Becker RC, Terrin M, Ross R, et al. Comparison of clinical outcomes for women and men after acute myocardial infarction. The Thrombolysis in Myocardial Infarction Investigators. Ann Intern Med 1994; 120:638–45.

34. Barzilay JI, Spiekerman CF, Wahl PW, et al. Cardiovascular disease

in older adults with glucose disorders: comparison of American Diabetes Association criteria for diabetes mellitus with WHO criteria. Lancet 1999; 354:622–5.

35. The DECODE study group. European Diabetes Epidemiology Group. Glucose tolerance and mortality: comparison of WHO and American Diabetes Association diagnostic criteria. Diabetes Epidemiology: Collaborative analysis Of Diagnostic criteria in Europe. Lancet 1999; 354: 617–21.

36. de Vegt F, Dekker JM, Ruhe HG, et al. Hyperglycaemia is associated with all-cause and cardiovascular mortality in the Hoorn population: the Hoorn Study. Diabetologia 1999; 42:926–31.

37. Malmberg K. Prospective randomised study of intensive insulin treatment on long term survival after acute myocardial infarction in patients with diabetes mellitus. DIGAMI (Diabetes Mellitus, Insulin–Glucose Infusion in Acute Myocardial Infarction) Study Group. Br Med J 1997; 314: 1512–15.

38. Capes SE, Hunt D, Malmberg K, Gerstein HC. Stress hyperglycaemia and increased risk of death after myocardial infarction in patients with and without diabetes: a systematic overview. Lancet 2000; 355:773–8.

39. de Micheli A, Medrano GA, Villarreal A, Sodi-Pallares D. [Protective effect of glucose–insulin–potassium solutions in myocardial damage caused by emetine]. Arch Inst Cardiol Mex 1975; 45:469–86.

40. Fath-Ordoubadi F, Beatt KJ. Glucose–insulin–potassium therapy for treatment of acute myocardial infarction: an overview of randomized placebo-controlled trials. Circulation 1997; 96:1152–6.

41. Garn SM, Clark DC. Trends in fatness and the origins of obesity. Pediatrics 1976; 57:443–56.

42. Black D, James WPI, Besser GM. Obesity. J R Coll Physicians Lond 1983; 17:5–65

43. Deurenberg P, Westrate JA, Seidell J. Body mass index as a measure of body fatness:age- and sex-specific prediction formulas. Br J Nutr 1991; 65:105–14

44. Lapidus L, Bengtsson C, Larsson B, et al. Distribution of adipose tissue and risk of cardiovascular disease and death: a 12 year follow up of participants in the population study of women in Gothenburg, Sweden. Br Med J (Clin Res Ed) 1984; 289:1257–61.

45. Larsson B, Svardsudd K, Welin L, et al. Abdominal adipose tissue distribution, obesity, and risk of cardiovascular disease and death: 13 year follow up of participants in the study of men born in 1913. Br Med J (Clin Res Ed) 1984; 288:1401-4.

46. WHO. The Asia-Pacific perspective: redefining obesity and its treatment. Geneva: WHO; 2000.

47. Hubert HB, Feinleib M, McNamara PM, Castelli WP. Obesity as an independent risk factor for cardiovascular disease: a 26-year follow-up of participants in the Framingham Heart Study. Circulation 1983; 67:968–77.

48. Manson JE, Willett WC, Stampfer MJ, et al. Body weight and mortality among women. New Engl J Med 1995; 333:677–85.

49. Must A, Jacques PF, Dallal GE, et al. H. Long-term morbidity and mortality of overweight adolescents. A follow-up of the Harvard Growth Study of 1922 to 1935. New Engl J Med 1992; 327: 1350–5.

50. Gunnell DJ, Frankel SJ, Nanchahal K, et al. Childhood obesity and adult cardiovascular mortality: a 57-y follow-up study based

on the Boyd Orr cohort. Am J Clin Nutr 1998; 67:1111–18.

51. Stevens J, Cai J, Pamuk ER, et al. The effect of age on the association between body-mass index and mortality. New Engl J Med 1998; 338:1–7.

52. Willett WC, Manson JE, Stampfer MJ, et al. Weight, weight change, and coronary heart disease in women. Risk within the 'normal' weight range. J Am Med Ass 1995; 273:461–5.

53. Ashton WD, Nanchahal K, Wood DA. Body mass index and metabolic risk factors for coronary heart disease in women. Eur Heart J 2001; 22:46–55.

54. Vague J. The degree of masculine differentiation of obesities, a factor determining predisposition to diabetes, atherosclerosis, gout and uric calculous disease. Am J Clin Nutr 1956; 4:20–34.

55. Bjorntorp P. 'Portal' adipose tissue as a generator of risk factors for cardiovascular disease and diabetes. Arteriosclerosis 1990; 10:493–6.

56. Alpert MA, Hashimi MW. Obesity and the heart. Am J Med Sci 1993; 306:117-23.

57. Messerli FH, Aepfelbacher FC. Hypertension and left-ventricular hypertrophy. Cardiol Clin 1995; 13:549–57.

58. Lavie CJ, Ventura HO, Messerli FH. Left ventricular hypertrophy. Its relationship to obesity and hypertension. Postgrad Med 1992; 91:131–2, 135–8, 141–3.

59. Duflou J, Virmani R, Rabin I, et al. Sudden death as a result of heart disease in morbid obesity. Am Heart J 1995; 130:306–13.

60. Frank S, Colliver JA, Frank A. The electrocardiogram in obesity: statistical analysis of 1,029 patients. J Am Coll Cardiol 1986; 7:295–9.

61. McKeigue PM, Shah B, Marmot MG. Relation of central obesity and insulin resistance with high diabetes prevalence and cardiovascular risk in South Asians. Lancet 1991; 337:382–6.

62. Charles MA, Eschwege E, Bennett PH. [Non-insulin-dependent diabetes in populations at risk: the Pima Indians]. Diabetes Metab 1997; 23 (Suppl 4):6–9.

63. Charles MA, Fontbonne A, Thibult N, et al. Risk factors for NIDDM in white population. Paris prospective study. Diabetes 1991; 40: 796–9.

64. Medalie JH, Papier C, Herman JB, et al. Diabetes mellitus among 10,000 adult men. I. Five-year incidence and associated variables. Isr J Med Sci 1974; 10: 681–97.

65. Harris MI. Impaired glucose tolerance in the U.S. population. Diabetes Care 1989; 12:464–74.

66. Van Itallie TB. Health implications of overweight and obesity in the United States. Ann Intern Med 1985; 103:983–8.

67. Colditz GA, Willett WC, Stampfer MJ, et al. Weight as a risk factor for clinical diabetes in women. Am J Epidemiol 1990; 132: 501–13.

68. Modan M, Karasik A, Halkin H, et al. Effect of past and concurrent body mass index on prevalence of glucose intolerance and type 2 (non-insulin-dependent) diabetes and on insulin response. The Israel study of glucose intolerance, obesity and hypertension. Diabetologia 1986; 29:82–9.

69. Jung RT. Obesity as a disease. Br Med Bull 1997; 53:307–21

70. Chan JM, Rimm EB, Colditz GA, et al. Obesity, fat distribution, and weight gain as risk factors for clinical diabetes in men. Diabetes Care 1994; 17:961–9.

71. Everhart JE, Pettitt DJ, Bennett PH, Knowler WC. Duration of

obesity increases the incidence of NIDDM. Diabetes 1992; 41: 235–40.

72. Austin MA, Selby JV. LDL subclass phenotypes and the risk factors of the insulin resistance syndrome. Int J Obes Relat Metab Disord 1995; 19(Suppl 1): S22–S26.

73. Ferrannini E, Camastra S. Relationship between impaired glucose tolerance, non-insulin-dependent diabetes mellitus and obesity. Eur J Clin Invest 1998; 28 (Suppl 2):3–6; discussion 6–7.

74. Carey VJ, Walters EE, Colditz GA, et al. Body fat distribution and risk of non-insulin-dependent diabetes mellitus in women. The Nurses' Health Study. Am J Epidemiol 1997; 145:614–19.

75. Despres JP. The insulin resistance-dyslipidemic syndrome of visceral obesity: effect on patients' risk. Obes Res 1998; 6(Suppl 1):8S–17S.

76. Despres JP, Lamarche B, Mauriege P, et al. Hyperinsulinemia as an independent risk factor for ischemic heart disease. New Engl J Med 1996; 334:952–7.

77. Bonadonna RC, Groop L, Kraemer N, et al. Obesity and insulin resistance in humans: a dose-response study. Metabolism 1990; 39:452–9.

78. Jensen MD, Haymond MW, Rizza RA, et al. Influence of body fat distribution on free fatty acid metabolism in obesity. J Clin Invest 1989; 83:1168–73.

79. Wiesenthal SR, Sandhu H, McCall RH, et al. Free fatty acids impair hepatic insulin extraction in vivo. Diabetes 1999; 48:766–74.

80. Rebrin K, Steil GM, Mittelman SD, Bergman RN. Causal linkage between insulin suppression of lipolysis and suppression of liver glucose output in dogs. J Clin Invest 1996; 98:741–9.

81. Boden G. Fatty acids and insulin resistance. Diabetes Care 1996; 19:394–5.

82. Hotamisligil GS, Shargill NS, Spiegelman BM. Adipose expression of tumor necrosis factor-alpha: direct role in obesity-linked insulin resistance. Science 1993; 259:87–91.

83. Hotamisligil GS, Johnson RS, Distel RJ, et al. Uncoupling of obesity from insulin resistance through a targeted mutation in aP2, the adipocyte fatty acid binding protein. Science 1996; 274:1377–9.

84. Hofmann C, Lorenz K, Braithwaite SS, et al. Altered gene expression for tumor necrosis factor-alpha and its receptors during drug and dietary modulation of insulin resistance. Endocrinology 1994; 134: 264–70.

85. Uysal KT, Wiesbrock SM, Marino MW, Hotamisligil GS. Protection from obesity-induced insulin resistance in mice lacking TNF-alpha function. Nature 1997; 389: 610-14.

86. Steppan CM, Bailey ST, Bhat S, et al. The hormone resistin links obesity to diabetes. Nature 2001; 409:307–12.

87. Haffner SM, Miettinen H. Insulin resistance implications for type II diabetes mellitus and coronary heart disease. Am J Med 1997; 103:152–62.

88. Vanhala MJ, Pitkajarvi TK, Kumpusalo EA, Takala JK. Obesity type and clustering of insulin resistance-associated cardiovascular risk factors in middle-aged men and women. Int J Obes Relat Metab Disord 1998; 22:369–74.

89. Lempiainen P, Mykkanen L, Pyorala K, et al. Insulin resistance syndrome predicts coronary heart disease events in elderly nondiabetic men. Circulation 1999; 100:123–8.

90. Ducimetiere P, Eschwege E, Papoz L, et al. Relationship of plasma insulin levels to the incidence of myocardial infarction and coronary heart disease mortality in a middle-aged population. Diabetologia 1980; 19:205–10.

91. Welborn TA, Wearne K. Coronary heart disease incidence and cardiovascular mortality in Busselton with reference to glucose and insulin concentrations. Diabetes Care 1979; 2:154–60.

92. Visser M, Bouter LM, McQuillan GM, et al. Elevated C-reactive protein levels in overweight and obese adults. J Am Med Ass 1999; 282:2131–5.

93. Ridker PM, Buring JE, Shih J, et al. Prospective study of C-reactive protein and the risk of future cardiovascular events among apparently healthy women. Circulation 1998; 98:731–3.

94. Ridker PM, Hennekens CH, Buring JE, Rifai N. C-reactive protein and other markers of inflammation in the prediction of cardiovascular disease in women. New Engl J Med 2000; 342:836–43.

95. Ford ES. Body mass index, diabetes, and C-reactive protein among U.S. adults. Diabetes Care 1999; 22:1971–7.

96. Vague P, Juhan-Vague I, Aillaud MF, et al. Correlation between blood fibrinolytic activity, plasminogen activator inhibitor level, plasma insulin level, and relative body weight in normal and obese subjects. Metabolism 1986; 35:250–3.

97. Erickson LA, Fici GJ, Lund JE, et al. Development of venous occlusions in mice transgenic for the plasminogen activator inhibitor-1 gene. Nature 1990; 346:74–6.

98. Hamsten A, Wiman B, de Faire U, Blomback M. Increased plasma levels of a rapid inhibitor of tissue plasminogen activator in young survivors of myocardial infarction. New Engl J Med 1985; 313:1557–63.

99. Hamsten A, de Faire U, Walldius G, et al. Plasminogen activator inhibitor in plasma: risk factor for recurrent myocardial infarction. Lancet 1987; 2:3–9.

100. Lupu F, Heim DA, Bachmann F, et al. Plasminogen activator expression in human atherosclerotic lesions. Arterioscler Thromb Vasc Biol 1995; 15:1444–55.

101. Sowers JR, Khoury S. Diabetes and hypertension: a review. Primary Care 1991; 18:509–24.

102. Sowers JR. Insulin and insulin-like growth factor in normal and pathological cardiovascular physiology. Hypertension 1997; 29:691–9.

103. Walsh MF, Dominguez LJ, Sowers JR. Metabolic abnormalities in cardiac ischemia. Cardiol Clin 1995; 13:529–38.

104. Stamler J, Vaccaro O, Neaton JD, Wentworth D. Diabetes, other risk factors, and 12-yr cardiovascular mortality for men screened in the Multiple Risk Factor Intervention Trial. Diabetes Care 1993; 16:434–44.

105. Modan M, Halkin H, Almog S, et al. Hyperinsulinemia. A link between hypertension obesity and glucose intolerance. J Clin Invest 1985; 75:809–17.

106. Stamler R, Stamler J, Riedlinger WF, et al. Weight and blood pressure. Findings in hypertension screening of 1 million Americans. J Am Med Ass 1978; 240:1607–10.

107. Friedman GD, Selby JV, Quesenberry CP, et al. Precursors of essential hypertension: body weight, alcohol and salt use, and parental history of hypertension. Prev Med 1988; 17:387–402.

108. Blair D, Habicht JP, Sims EA, et al. Evidence for an increased risk for hypertension with centrally

located body fat and the effect of race and sex on this risk. Am J Epidemiol 1984; 119:526–40.

109. Reisin E, Frohlich ED, Messerli FH, et al. Cardiovascular changes after weight reduction in obesity hypertension. Ann Intern Med 1983; 98:315–19.

110. Tuck ML, Sowers J, Dornfeld L, et al. The effect of weight reduction on blood pressure, plasma renin activity, and plasma aldosterone levels in obese patients. New Engl J Med 1981; 304:930–3.

111. Tuck ML. Role of salt in the control of blood pressure in obesity and diabetes mellitus. Hypertension 1991; 17:1135–42.

112. DeFronzo RA, Cooke CR, Andres R, et al. The effect of insulin on renal handling of sodium, potassium, calcium, and phosphate in man. J Clin Invest 1975; 55: 845–55.

113. Ward KD, Sparrow D, Landsberg L, et al. Influence of insulin, sympathetic nervous system activity, and obesity on blood pressure: the Normative Aging Study. J Hypertens 1996; 14:301–8.

114. Landsberg L. Role of the sympathetic adrenal system in the pathogenesis of the insulin resistance syndrome. Ann NY Acad Sci 1999; 892:84–90.

115. Hansson L, Zanchetti A, Carruthers SG, et al. Effects of intensive blood-pressure lowering and low-dose aspirin in patients with hypertension: principal results of the Hypertension Optimal Treatment (HOT) randomised trial. HOT Study Group. Lancet 1998; 351:1755–62.

116. Grundy SM, Barnett JP. Metabolic and health complications of obesity. Dis Mon 1990; 36:641–731.

117. Barrett-Connor E, Grundy SM, Holdbrook MJ. Plasma lipids and diabetes mellitus in an adult community. Am J Epidemiol 1982; 115:657–63.

118. Fontbonne A, Eschwege E, Cambien F, et al. Hypertriglyceridaemia as a risk factor of coronary heart disease mortality in subjects with impaired glucose tolerance or diabetes. Results from the 11-year follow-up of the Paris Prospective Study. Diabetologia 1989; 32:300–4.

119. Lean ME, Powrie JK, Anderson AS, Garthwaite PH. Obesity, weight loss and prognosis in type 2 diabetes. Diabet Med 1990; 7:228–33.

120. Hanefeld M, Fischer S, Schmechel H, et al. Diabetes Intervention Study. Multi-intervention trial in newly diagnosed NIDDM. Diabetes Care 1991; 14: 308–17.

121. Goldstein DJ. Beneficial health effects of modest weight loss. Int J Obes Relat Metab Disord 1992; 16:397–415.

122. Wilding J, Williams G. Diabetes and obesity. In: Kopelman PG, (editor). Clinical obesity. Oxford: Blackwell Science; 1998: 308–49.

3

Hypertension and diabetes: what do recent trials tell us?

Paul M Dodson

Introduction

The frequent co-occurrence of hypertension in Type 2 diabetes is well recognized, with the prevalence of hypertension in subjects with Type 2 diabetes almost twice that of the non-diabetic population.[1] Hypertension not only exaggerates the high risk of widespread atherosclerotic vascular disease in diabetic subjects but also increases the risk of microvascular complications.[2] In diabetic subjects, systolic hypertension is firmly established as a risk factor for cardiovascular disease.[2,3] For example, the UK Prospective Diabetes Study (UKPDS) has recently demonstrated a 15% increase in coronary artery disease per 10mmHg rise in systolic blood pressure.[2] In microvascular disease, increasing systemic blood pressure and hypertension are the single most important risk factors for progression of diabetic nephropathy, such that diabetic patients with nephropathy have a > 80% prevalence of hypertension, 40% in those with microalbuminuria and 20% in those with normoalbuminuria.[4] Recent studies have confirmed that hypertension is a significant risk factor for diabetic retinopathy, with a strong association between hypertension and increasing hard exudates, haemorrhages, and other severe forms of retinopathy (e.g. maculopathy, proliferative retinopathy and retino-vascular disease).[5]

The beneficial effects of antihypertensive therapy in non-diabetic populations are well established. For example, the Systolic Hypertension in the Elderly Programme (SHEP) study showed that, over 5 years of treatment, reduction of systolic blood pressure with a thiazide, beta (β)-blocking drug or reserpine from a mean of 155mmHg to 143mmHg reduced major cardiovascular events by 55 per 1000 patients treated.[6] The Systolic Hypertension in Europe trial (SYST-Eur) has further confirmed this finding using the calcium antagonist nitrendepine.[6] Findings in these and other landmark hypertension treatment trials have allowed recent updates of guidelines on the management of hypertension that have been published by national and international societies.[7,8]

Until the new trial evidence was reported from the large randomized trials from 1998 onwards, the assumption had been that the beneficial effects of treatment of hypertension could be extrapolated from the non-diabetic treatment trials to the diabetic population. Evidence of benefit of treatment of hypertension was only available prior to 1998 in patients with diabetic nephropathy. There was no evidence that the use of antihypertensive therapy in the diabetic population attenuated the risk of microvascular or macrovascular complications in Type 2 diabetes. Indeed, much of the evidence for the reduction of microvascular disease has been extrapolated from the work done in Type 1 diabetes, e.g. with diabetic nephropathy.[1,4,9] There were also concerns that certain classes of antihypertensive agents could adversely affect the outcome in patients with Type 2 diabetes due to worsening of other metabolic factors, in particular glycaemia and dyslipidaemia. Furthermore, the threshold level at which to treat hypertension in diabetes had not been established. This chapter will therefore review the recent trial data for treatment of hypertension in Type 2 diabetic subjects (but applicable to both Type 1 and Type 2 diabetes), and highlight the conclusions that can been made that will influence current management. More trials are ongoing and future prospects will be discussed.

Trial evidence

A number of recently published, large hypertension trials have included substantial numbers of patients with diabetes, allowing separate subgroup analyses to be conducted on diabetic patients with hypertension.[10] These trials have shown specific effects in patients with coexistent diabetes and hypertension. Indeed, it is fortunate that subgroups of patients with diabetes were included in the trial as, in two of these, the results in diabetics showed the most persuasive reason for treatment of hypertension [e.g. the Hypertension Optimal Treatment (HOT) and Captopril Prevention Project (CAPPP) studies].[10] A summary of the results of the six major randomized controlled trials, including large numbers of patients with Type 2 diabetes, are shown in Table 3.1.

Does antihypertensive therapy reduce mortality, morbidity and microvascular end-points in Type 1 diabetic patients?

The initial studies in Type 1 diabetic patients focused on diabetic nephropathy. The first reports clearly demonstrated that lowering blood pressure in patients with established diabetic nephropathy reduced the progression of decline in renal function of patients with diabetic nephropathy, and that angiotensin-converting-enzyme (ACE) inhibitors have a renoprotective effect.[4,9] The benefit of hypertension treatment, and specifically with ACE inhibitors, were also demonstrated in patients with chronic renal failure.[11]

Interest has recently focused on the possibility of treating patients at an early stage of diabetic nephropathy in order to stop its progression. Incipient nephropathy may last for up to 15 years before it progresses to overt nephropathy, though c. 60% of patients with microalbuminuria may never progress that far.[9] A number of studies has suggested that treatment of blood pressure in incipient nephropathy does indeed delay progression. Large prospective studies have shown that antihypertensive therapy with ACE inhibitors in patients with microalbuminuria appears to protect against the development of overt nephropathy.[12] In one multicentre double-blind randomized parallel group study, 335 patients with Type 2 diabetes and microalbuminuria were studied over a 1-year period, following random allocation to treatment with either lisinopril or nifedipine.[13] A significant reduction in urine and albumin excretion was observed in the lisinopril-treated group. The Melbourne Nephropathy Study Group examined 43 patients with microalbuminuria and found that treatment of blood pressure with either perindopril or nifedipine caused a reduction in the progressive rise of albumin excretion rate after 1 year, with no significant difference in efficacy between the two treatment groups.[4] Recently, the Eurodiab Controlled Trial of Lisinopril in Insulin-dependent Diabetes (EUCLID) study, using a randomized double-blind placebo-controlled design, evaluated the effect of treatment with lisinopril versus placebo on the progression of albumin excretion rate in 440 normotensive normoalbuminuric patients with Type 2 diabetes.[14] After 2 years the absolute treatment difference between the two groups, in the absence of significant changes in blood pressure, was $1\mu g$/minute (a reduction of 12.7%). Although this effect was not statistically significant, it may be of clinical importance in limiting the development of renal disease, thereby reducing the proportion of patients who would ultimately require renal replacement therapy. This latter study supports the notion that patients with microalbuminuria, either normotensive or hypertensive, should be treated with antihypertensive therapy, in particular ACE inhibitors.

A recent meta-analysis of the 12 trials of 698 patients studied with microalbuminuria suggests that ACE inhibitors significantly reduce the progression to macroalbuminuria and increases the chance of regression.[15] Beneficial effects were weaker at the lowest levels of microalbuminuria but did not differ according to other baseline risk factors.[4] Importantly, changes in blood pressure could not entirely explain the antiproteinuric effect of ACE inhibition. A few long-term studies with other agents have been reported, principally with calcium-channel blockers, to assess the effects on progression of diabetic nephropathy either alone or in combination with ACE inhibitors. Those studies suggest that that the non-dihydropyridine calcium-channel blockers (e.g. diltiazem- and vera-

Table 3.1 Recent randomized, controlled trials of hypertension-related treatments in subjects with diabetes.

Trial	Patients (n)	Follow-up (years)	Treatment	Fall in blood pressure (mmHg)	Reduction in end-points summary	Implication?
SHEP	583	5	Thiazide and β-blocker	9.8/2.2	All cardiovascular disease events (46–66%)	Thiazides and β-blockers effective
UKPDS	1148	9	Captopril or atenolol	10/5	Strokes (44%), diabetes-related deaths (32%), microvascular end-points (37%)	Target blood pressure achieved < 40/85mmHg; cost-effective; microvascular event reduction; no apparent difference between ACE inhibitors and β-blockers
HOT	1501	4	Calcium antagonist	29.9/24.4	Major cardiovascular events and total mortality (50%)	Target < 140/85mmHg; two or more agents commonly required; safety of calcium antagonists confirmed
SYST-Eur	492	2	Calcium antagonist	10.11/4.5	All major cardiovascular events (41–70%)	Calcium antagonists safe and effective; impressive reductions in mortality
CAPPP	552	6	Captopril versus β-blocker or thiazide	Both 16/10	Captopril group reduced fatal and non-fatal MI by 34%	Suggests effectiveness of ACE inhibition

Trial	n	Duration (years)	Intervention		Outcome	Conclusion
MICRO-HOPE	3577	4.5	ACE inhibition in high-risk subjects	2.4/1.0[a]	Total mortality (−24%), MI (−22%), stroke (−33%), microvascular (−16%)	Benefit even in normotensive patients (42%); ACE inhibition safe and effective; treat those with microvascular disease (particularly early nephropathy)
EUCLID	530	2	ACE inhibition	3/2[a]	Progression of retinopathy	ACE inhibition may have a specific retinoprotective effect
STENO II	160	3.8	ACE inhibition; tight glycaemic and lipid control		Less progression to macroalbuminuria (27%) and retinopathy (45%)	Multifactorial intervention

All the trials included patients with Type 2 diabetes except EUCLID, which included normotensive patients with Type 1 diabetes.
SHEP, Systolic Hypertension in the Elderly Program; UKPDS, UK Prospective Diabetes Study; HOT Hypertension Optimal Treatment; SYST-Eur, Systolic Hypertension in Europe Study; CAPP, Captopril Prevention Project; MICRO-HOPE, Microalbuminuria, Cardiovascular, and Renal Outcomes in the Heart Outcomes Prevention Evaluation; EUCLID, Eurodiab Controlled Trial of Lisinopril in Insulin-dependent Diabetes; ACE, angiotensin-converting enzyme; MI, myocardial infarction.
a Many patients normotensive at entry.

pamil-like agents) appear to reduce proteinuria more effectively than do the dihydropyridine agents, even in the presence of similar blood pressure control.[4,9]

The angiotensin II antagonists are relatively a new class of agent which specifically block the effect of angiotensin II at the receptor (Type 1) site.[16,17] There is current data to show that these agents may be as effective as ACE inhibitors in delaying the progression of renal injury in animal models. In humans, small clinical studies have demonstrated improvement in markers of renal protection compared with calcium antagonists. There are several studies under way using a range of angiotensin II antagonists in patients with Type 1 diabetes to determine whether or not they are as effective as ACE inhibitors in renal and retinopathy protection in humans. The recent Candesartan and Lisinopril Microalbuminuria (CALM) report has demonstrated the safety and efficacy of a combination of an ACE inhibitor with an angiotensin II receptor blocker, with similar effects on urine protein excretion.[18] The combination resulted in an 8mmHg greater reduction in systolic pressure when compared to the single agent alone.[1,7]

There is a suggestion that in Type 1 diabetic subjects antihypertensive drugs could be of benefit in patients with established diabetic retinopathy.[11] The EUCLID study involved randomization of predominately normotensive, normoalbuminuric Type 1 diabetic patients to placebo (N = 166) or an ACE inhibitor (N = 159).[19] At 2 years, ACE inhibition was associated with a statistically significant (50%) reduction in the progression of retinopathy by at least one Eurodiab level (p = < 0.02) and the odds ratio for proliferative retinopathy was 0.18 with lisinopril treatment (p = < 0.03) This effect could not be wholly accounted for by the 3mmHg reduction in diastolic pressure in the lisinopril-treated group. However, caution has been applied to the study since there were differences in glycated haemoglobin between the placebo- and the lisinopril-treated groups. Nevertheless, meta-analysis of other studies of ACE inhibitors in normotensive diabetics have also shown evidence of a beneficial effect on retinopathy.

The most favourable results in Type 1 diabetic patients suggest than antihypertensive treatment may delay progression from normal glomerular filtration rates to end-stage renal disease by up to 30 years, rather than the average 7 years in inadequately treated patients.[4,9,11,12] Many studies have helped to establish target blood pressure levels for patients with diabetic nephropathy – < 130/80mmHg but preferably 125/75mmHg (see Table 3.2). Retrospective studies in Type 1 diabetic patients suggest a reduction in accumulative death rate over the past 20 years of antihypertensive treatment from 80% to < 20% at 10 years in patients with overt diabetic nephropathy.[4,9] However, in Type 1 diabetic patients without nephropathy there are no randomized controlled trials focusing on cardiovascular end-points (i.e. prevention of stroke, myocardial infarction and peripheral vascular disease).

Table 3.2 British Hypertension Society guidelines on treating hypertension patients with diabetes.[7]

	Type 1 diabetes		Type 2 diabetes	
	Without nephropathy	With nephropathy	Without nephropathy	With nephropathy
Threshold for treatment (mmHg)	≥140/90	≥140/90	≥140/90	≥140/90
Target blood pressure (mmHg)	<140/80	<130/80[a]	<140/80	<130/85[a]

[a]Target blood pressure < 125/75mmHg, if proteinuria > 1g/day.

Is antihypertensive therapy of benefit in Type 2 diabetic patients?

A number of recently published, large hypertension trials have included substantial numbers of patients with diabetes, allowing separate sub-group analysis to be conducted on Type 2 diabetic patients with hypertension.[10] These trials have shown specific effects in patients that are coexistent with diabetes and hypertension. Indeed, it is fortunate that subgroups of patients with diabetes were included in the trials as, in two of these, the results in diabetics showed the most benefit of treatment of hypertension (the HOT and CAPPP studies).[10] (A summary of the details and findings of the six large randomized prospective trials are shown in Table 3.1.) The key studies include SHEP,[6] UKPDS,[20] HOT,[21] SYST-Eur,[22] Heart Outcomes Prevention Evaluation (HOPE)[23] and CAPPP.[24] Eight thousand Type 2 diabetic patients have been randomized in these trials, using the four principle classes of antihypertensive therapeutic agents, i.e. thiazides, beta (β) blockers, ACE inhibitors and calcium antagonists. Overall, cardiovascular disease events were reduced in hypertensive Type 2 diabetics by 22–70%, with antihypertensive therapy over treatment periods arranging from 2 to 9 years.[10]

Does antihypertensive therapy reduce mortality and morbidity in Type 2 diabetics?

Analysis of the subgroup of diabetic patients who formed part of the SHEP study has been reported.[6] This included 583 elderly diabetic subjects who were treated with chlorthalidone, with and without atenolol or reserpine, compared to placebo. In the tight blood pressure control group, the reduction of systolic blood pressure was 9.8mmHg lower than the less tight blood pressure control group. There was an impressive reduction of relative risk of myocardial infarction by 54%. These findings were confirmed and extended by the UKPDS and HOT studies.[20,21] The UKPDS set out to determine whether tight glycaemic control could reduce adverse complications in subjects with Type 2 diabetes, but embedded in a factorial design in the original UKPDS cohort, a multicentre randomized control trial of tight versus less tight blood pressure control was undertaken. The less tight control group (n = 390) was treated with antihypertensive drugs avoiding ACE inhibitors or β-blockers. The tight control group was further randomized to either captopril or atenolol, and other drugs were added if control was inadequate. Medium follow-up was 8.4 years and mean blood pressure in the tight control group was 10/5mmHg lower than the less tight group, achieving a mean blood pressure of 144/82mmHg. After 9 years follow-up a 32% reduction in diabetes-related deaths, a 44% reduction in strokes and a 34% reduction in combined macrovascular end-points was seen. These results thus provide firm evidence that tight blood pressure control is beneficial in patients with Type 2 diabetes. Twenty-nine per cent of patients needed three or more antihypertensive therapies to lower their blood pressure to target values. Analysis of cost effectiveness of tight blood pressure control in hypertensive Type 2 diabetic patients has shown very good value at £720.00 per life year gained. Interestingly, the UKPDS demonstrated that the benefit of reducing blood pressure in patients with Type 2 diabetes was much greater than the benefit of improving glycaemic control, which appeared to influence microvascular more than macrovascular complications.

The SYST-Eur trial, studying 492 diabetic hypertensive patients, showed similar to more impressive benefits of blood pressure reduction as those achieved in the UKPDS trial.[22] Treatment of systolic hypertension in the elderly diabetic subjects in this trial reduced total mortality by 55%, cardiovascular mortality by 76%, cardiovascular end-points by 69% and an overall reduction of 73%. These large reductions were achieved over a 2 year follow-up period with calcium antagonists therapy of nitrendipine.

The CAPPP study included a subgroup of 572 patients with Type 2 diabetes who were allocated to receive either captopril or conventional therapy, to ascertain whether a diastolic pressure of < 90mmHg could be achieved.[24] While there was no significant difference between the conventional and captopril treatment in patients without diabetes, in the subgroup with diabetes, captopril was associated with a significant reduction in myocardial infarction by 34% and all cardiac events by 67%. The recent Microalbuminuria Cardiovascular, and Renal Outcomes in the Heart Outcomes Prevention Evaluation (MICRO-HOPE) study has provided further strong evidence of the benefit of treatment with ACE inhibition in a large Type 2 diabetic population.[23] Rather than focusing on hypertension, this trial examined the hypothesis that ACE inhibition with ramipril would reduce cardiovascular events in a group of patients who were at high risk of future cardiovascular disease but who would not normally be treated with ACE inhibitors as they had no clinical evidence of left ventricular dysfunction. Patients either had documented cardiovascular disease (with definite coronary artery disease), peripheral vascular disease or stroke, or diabetes and one other cardiovascular risk factor (e.g. total cholesterol > 5.2mmol, high-density lipoprotein cholesterol (HDL-C) < 0.9mmol, hypertension, microalbuminuria or cigarette smoking). There were 3577 diabetic patients included in the study, which was halted 6 months prematurely by the data and safety monitoring board because of significant and repeated benefit from ramipril. The trial had a mean follow-up of 4.5 years. Ramipril treatment was associated with risk reductions of myocardial infarction by 22%, stroke by 33%, cardiovascular deaths by 37% and total mortality by 24% compared with placebo. There were also findings with regard to combined microvascular endpoints that will be discussed later.

Does treatment of hypertension reduce microvascular complications in Type 2 diabetes?

This important question has been addressed in both the UKPDS and the MICRO-HOPE Studies.[20,23] In the UKPDS study, retinopathy was defined as the presence of one microaneurysm in one eye or worse, using retinal photography, with progression defined as a two-step change in the modified Early Treatment of Diabetic Retinopathy Study (ETDRS) grade. Albuminuria was assessed using spot clinic urine albumin concentrations and the development of neuropathy by loss of both ankle or knee reflexes, or changes on biothesiometer readings. Overall, the tight blood pressure control group had a 37% reduction in microvascular disease compared to the less tight control group. This effect was predominantly due to a reduction in either the development or progression of retinopathy. The tight control group had a 34% reduction in the risk of retinal photocoagulation (mainly for maculopathy) and a 47% lower risk of reduction in visual acuity. In contrast, there was no significant reduction in the risk of microalbuminuria or macroalbuminuria over a 9 year follow-up between the tight and less tight blood pressure control groups. However, there was a trend for lower rates of clinical proteinuria in patients treated with captopril compared to those on atenolol. There was no significant difference in the development of neuropathy between the tight versus the less tight blood pressure control groups.

One third of the study population in the MICRO-HOPE study had microalbuminuria at entry. ACE inhibitor treatment (ramipril) reduced the development of overt nephropathy, confirming the results of smaller studies in Type 2 diabetic subjects. The risk of developing microalbuminuria was also reduced in patients who were normoalbuminuric on entry into the trial. With regard to retinopathy, there was a reduction in laser therapy requirement in those treated with ACE inhibition by 22% when compared to placebo but this did not reach statistical significance. When the microvascular end-points were combined, both renal and retinal, there was an overall 16% reduction, which was statistically significant.

It would therefore appear that treatment of hypertension in Type 2 diabetic subjects does have benefit in reduction of microvascular end-points in these two randomized controlled trials. Supporting data is also provided for this concept by the small STENO Type 2 trial that reported a 45% reduction in the progression of retinopathy on an intensive treatment regime, including ACE inhibition, over a 3.8-year period.[25]

What is the threshold of treatment and target blood pressure for Type 2 hypertensive diabetics?

The recent hypertension trials have allowed the calculation of both target and threshold blood pressure for treatment in diabetic subjects. Concern had previously been expressed that excessive lowering of blood pressure could lead to an increase in cardiovascular mortality rather than a reduction – the so-called J-shaped curve. The important results of the HOT trial have shed light on this.[21] This trial enrolled nearly 19,000 hypertensive patients and included 1501 diabetic subjects. Patients were randomized to target diastolic pressures of < 90, < 85 or < 80mmHg. In addition, half the subjects in each arm were randomized to receive aspirin. Treatment commenced with felodopine, a long-acting calcium antagonist, and additional antihypertensive therapy was added to achieve target diastolic pressure. Blood pressure reduction > 20mmHg was achieved in the great majority of patients, which required at least two antihypertensive agents in 60% of the patients. In the diabetic subjects the lowest incidence of major cardiovascular events occurred when a mean systolic pressure of 138.5mmHg and a mean diastolic pressure of 83mmHg were achieved. Further reduction in blood pressure below these levels was not associated with increased benefit, but equally was not associated with increased mortality and was therefore reassuring with regard to the J-shaped hypothesis. In addition, this study was the first to demonstrate, in primary prevention in diabetic subjects, that addition of aspirin to antihypertensive therapy reduces cardiovascular events by a further 15%.

The findings of the HOT study are complimentary and support those of the UKPDS, which has shown added benefit in intensifying blood pressure control in diabetic subjects.[21] Achieving a blood pressure of 144/82mmHg or less reduced diabetes-related deaths and cardiovascular end-points. Therefore, together these studies suggest a target blood pressure of 140mmHg systolic and 80mmHg diastolic or less; these values are now accepted and adopted in most national and international guidelines for treatment for hypertension (see Table 3.2).[7]

Which antihypertensive drugs should be used in diabetic subjects?

Early trials of antihypertensive therapy in hypertensive subjects have commonly used thiazide diuretics, β-blocking agents and other older drugs as the first- or second-line therapy. It has been suggested that these agents may be disadvantageous in diabetic subjects with hypertension due to the increased risk of deterioration in other metabolic factors.[26] The newer ACE inhibitors and calcium-channel blockers appear to be metabolically neutral and may therefore be of greater potential benefit.[27] The efficacy of these newer agents has now been extensively studied in a number of recent trials. Previous reports of adverse effects of calcium-channel blockers on mortality, morbidity and cancer rates in non-diabetic subjects had caused considerable concern.[10] The hypothesis that calcium-channel blockade might increase cardiovascular mortality was supported by three early large studies involving diabetic patients. These were the Appropriate Blood Pressure Control in Diabetes (ABCD) Trial,[28] the Fosinopril Versus Amlodipine Cardiovascular Events Randomized Trial (FACET)[29] and the Multicentre Isradipine Diuretic Atherosclerosis Study (MIDAS).[30] Two of these trials were comparing ACE inhibitors to calcium antagonists. Part of the explanation for the difference in rates of myocardial infarction between the groups may be due to the ACE inhibitor being particularly beneficial and not the calcium antagonist being harmful. MIDAS suggested a significantly greater number of cardiovascular events in the calcium-channel-treated group compared to diuretic therapy, but this observation was only based on the small number of a total 21 events over 3 years.

The publication of the large SYST-Eur has been reassuring and has confirmed the benefit of the calcium antagonist therapy with regard to cardiovascular events.[22] The principle results of this diabetic subgroup analysis demonstrated that calcium antagonist-based therapy led to impressive reductions of 55% in total mortality, 76% in cardiovascular mortality and 73% in strokes, as compared with placebo. The cancer rate was lower in the calcium-channel-treated group. Further evidence that calcium antagonist therapy is not harmful in diabetic subjects was given by the results of the HOT trial (see previous description).

These studies therefore provide considerable reassurance for clinicians caring for diabetic subjects. Whilst it seems likely that ACE inhibitor drugs may be more beneficial than calcium antagonists, there is little doubt that the latter drugs are also protective against cardiovascular disease in diabetic subjects with systolic hypertension.

Both SHEP and UKPDS have provided data using thiazides and β-blocking agents, and comparisons with newer ACE inhibitors.[22,31] Five hundred and eighty-three elderly subjects were included in the placebo-controlled SHEP study, where patients were allocated to receive treatment with chlorthalidone, with or without atenolol or reserpine.[14] The results showed a reduction in systolic pressure that was 9.8mmHg lower than that of the control group and a reduction in the relative risk of myocardial infarction by 46%. This is a reassuring finding in view of the potential adverse effects of β blockers and thiazides in patients with diabetes. The UKPDS study of hypertension in diabetes compared the use of ACE inhibitor drugs with β-blocking agents.[31] Of the 758 patients allocated to tight blood pressure control, 400 were allocated to captopril and 358 to atenolol. Both drugs were equally effective in reducing blood pressure and in reducing cardiovascular end-points. However, it should be noted that many more patients receiving atenolol (35%) stopped the therapy before the end of the study compared to those on captopril (22%); this was due to side effects.

There is increasing data available on the benefit of ACE inhibition in patients with diabetes from the point of view of both renal and cardiovascular protection. In the CAPPP study, a subgroup of 572 patients with diabetes was allocated to receive either captopril or conventional therapy to ascertain whether a diastolic pressure of < 90mmHg could be achieved.[24] Whilst there is no significant difference between conventional and captopril in patients without diabetes, in the subgroup of diabetic patients, captopril treatment was associated with a significant reduction in myocardial infarction (−34%) and all cardiac events (−67%). The recent HOPE study, which lasted 4.5 years, assessed the role of ACE inhibition in patients at high risk of cardiovascular events.[23] A total of 3577 patients with diabetes were included. Patients were at least 55 years old and the patients with diabetes had at least one other cardiovascular risk factor or a history of previous cardiovascular events. Patients were randomly allocated to receive placebo or ACE inhibition therapy. In this group of diabetic subjects, ramipril treatment was associated with risk reduction of myocardial infarction (22%), stroke (33%), cardiovascular deaths (37%) and total mortality (24%) compared with placebo. The CAPPP and HOPE studies have therefore confirmed the impressive benefit of ACE inhibition therapy in patients with diabetes in terms of cardiovascular disease.[23,24]

Whilst there is no large randomized trial studying ACE inhibitors in Type 1 diabetics with regard to cardiovascular outcome, the proven renal protective effect has led to ACE inhibitors being the drug of choice for Type 1 diabetic subjects with hypertension.[4,9,14] For Type 2 diabetics, the large trials described previously have confirmed the benefit in terms of cardiovascular outcome of four groups of antihypertensive drugs, i.e. thiazide diuretics, β-blockers, calcium-channel blockers and ACE inhibitors. In the past, there has been much discussion as to the choice of first-line antihypertensive agents for diabetic subjects. There is broad agreement that ACE inhibitors are a first choice, but as at least 60% of diabetic patients with hypertension will require at least two agents or more, current emphasis will be on combination therapies. The ability to use combination therapy at lower doses than would be required in monotherapy lessens the potential for side effects and should have an additive/synergistic effect. The latter is of major importance, particularly in Type 2 diabetic patients who already face the prospect of multiple therapies, including oral hypoglycaemic, statin and aspirin treatment. Logical combinations include a thiazide diuretic and an ACE inhibitor, a calcium-channel blocker and an ACE inhibitor, and a thiazide and a β-blocker. There are only a limited number of fixed combination therapies currently available in the UK but it is envisaged that more will become available. A new potential combination has been demonstrated in the recent CALM study, which demonstrated safety and efficacy of the combination of an ACE inhibitor (lisinopril) with an angiotensin II receptor blocker (candesartan).[18] The combination resulted in an 8mmHg greater reduction in systolic pressure when compared to the single agent alone.

Questions not answered by the recent trials

The recent studies do suggest that the newer drugs, such as ACE inhibitors and calcium antagonists, are safe and effective in patients with Type 2 diabetes. However, a number questions remain unanswered (see Table 3.3). The role of the newer antihypertensive agents, such as angiotensin II receptor antagonists, in diabetic patients is as yet unclear. These drugs appear to have good efficacy and side-effect profiles, and are metabolically neutral.[32] They should have theoretical benefits in patients with nephropathy. Alpha (α) blockers also appear to be metabolically neutral and may be of benefit in diabetic patients.[33] The role of α-blockers and angiotensin II antagonists is being elucidated by the ongoing Antihypertensive and Lipid Lowering Treatment to Prevent Heart Attack Trial (ALLHAT).[33] However, following an interim analysis of the study, the α-blocker arm has been stopped prematurely, as this treatment was associated with a 1.25-fold increase in the relative risk of combined cardiovascular disease end-points when compared with thiazide diuretic treatment. This difference was mainly related to an increase in the relative risks of heart failure and stroke.[34] Their role in diabetic patients with hypertension is as an add-on therapy.

Remaining issues include some controversy as to whether or not ACE inhibitors, particularly in Type 2 diabetes, are superior to other agents in slowing the progression of diabetic nephropathy. There are also no randomized, controlled trials focusing on cardiovascular end-points in Type 1 diabetic subjects.

More work needs to be done in terms of diabetic retinopathy, especially to elucidate whether or not ACE inhibitors have a specific effect on delaying presentation and progression of retinopathy over and above

Table 3.3 Conclusions and questions.

Conclusions drawn from the recent trials of hypertension in diabetes
- Treating hypertension reduces mortality in patients with diabetes and the effect is much greater than that seen in non-diabetic patients
- Treating hypertension reduces retinopathy and loss of visual acuity in patients with diabetes
- Treating hypertension is more cost-effective than improving glycaemic control in patients with diabetes
- The threshold for treatment of blood pressure in patients with diabetes is ≥140/90mmHg
- Calcium antagonists and thiazide diuretics are effective in reducing mortality and morbidity in hypertensive patients with diabetes
- ACE inhibitors and β-blockers are safe and equally effective in patients with diabetes, and probably reduce mortality and morbidity
- Most patients with hypertension and diabetes require more than one antihypertensive agent to control blood pressure

Questions not yet answered by the recent studies
- What is the target for treatment of hypertension in patients with diabetes? Is aiming for ≤140/80mmHg adequate?
- Does lower target blood pressure reduce mortality further?
- Should all hypertensive patients with diabetes be treated with aspirin?
- What is the role of other classes of antihypertensive agents such as α-blockers and angiotensin II receptor antagonists?
- Should thresholds and targets for treatment be lower in patients with microvascular disease?
- Should microalbuminuric Type 2 diabetic patients be treated with ACE inhibitors irrespective of blood pressure?

their blood pressure lowering effects.[5] In addition, angiotensin II antagonists have been suggested to have a similar role to ACE inhibitors and studies are underway to analyse this.

Consideration of non-pharmacological therapy has not been included in recent treatment trials, although this remains an important adjunct to therapy. This is particularly relevant because of the multiple drug therapies commonly needed to achieve blood pressure targets, and other target such as glucose, glycated haemoglobin and low-density lipoprotein cholesterol, HDL-C and total cholesterol levels.

Modern diabetic management and therapy will now include strategies for glycaemic control, lipid lowering, antiplatelet drug therapy and blood pressure control. There is, however, little evidence that this multifactorial intervention is of benefit in terms of cardiovascular outcome, nor in microvascular end-points. Although, in the small Steno Type 2 study, conventional treatment was compared with intensified treatment and antihypertensive therapy – ACE inhibition, aspirin and lipid lowering with statins. In the 159 patients randomized and followed up over 3.8 years, the intensively treated patients had significantly less progression to microalbuminuria, retinopathy and autonomic neuropathy. This study was not efficiently powered to assess cardiovascular end-points.

Implications for clinical practice and the future

Table 3.4 and Figure 3.1 summarize some of the conclusions drawn and the questions remaining from the recent clinical trials in hypertensive patients with diabetes. More trial data is still to come, in particular the ALLHAT and Anglo-Scandinavian Cardiac Outcomes Trial (ASCOT) studies that will give valuable information in large cohorts of hypertensive diabetic subjects (see Table 3.5). The results of recent meta-analysis of the hypertensive treatment trials has suggested that more attention should be focused on systolic rather than diastolic blood pressure.[3] A systolic pressure of 140mmHg appears to be the key value for hypertension management, both the threshold value for intervention and the treatment goal.[35] There should also be an increased role for ambulatory blood pressure monitoring.[36] The abolition of the mercury sphygmomanometer for electronic blood pressure devices, which can also be used for home blood pressure recording, should have more widespread usage.[37] A single electronic device that allows measurement of blood glucose and blood pressure should be highly desirable for patients with diabetes.

Table 3.4 Principal findings of the treatment trials of diabetes and hypertension.

Type 2 diabetes hypertension treatment
- Reduces cardiovascular morbidity and mortality (evidence for thiazides, β-blockers, ACE inhibitors and calcium antagonists)
- The threshold for intervention is ⩾140/90mmHg, with a target of ⩾140/80mmHg
- More than 60% of patients will require two or more agents to achieve target blood pressure threshold
- Patient quality of life is not reduced and treatment is cost-effective
- Reduces progression of diabetic nephropathy
- Reduces progression of retinopathy and loss of visual acuity

Type 1 diabetes hypertension treatment
- Has not been shown to reduce cardiovascular end-points
- Reduces progression of nephropathy in the incipient and overt phases
- The threshold for intervention is ⩾140/90mmHg, with a target of <130/80mmHg
- ACE inhibition has a specific renoprotective effect and may delay progression of retinopathy
- ACE inhibitors are recommended as a first-line treatment

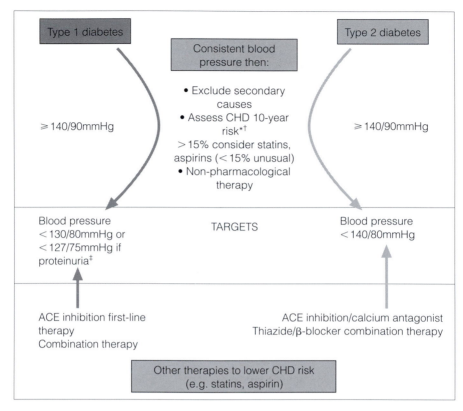

Figure 3.1

Management of hypertension associated with diabetes. *Coronary heart disease (CHD) risk calculated by the Framingham equation; †in the context of secondary prevention (i.e. existing CHD), statins (or fibrates) and aspirin are appropriate; ‡proteinuria > 1g/day. ACE, angiotensin-converting enzyme. Serum cholesterol target < 4.8mmol/l.

With the advent of randomized controlled trials examining large numbers of hypertensive patients with diabetes, indicating proven benefit in treating diabetic patients with hypertension, the evidence base is now available to encourage all clinicians to make a significant impact on cardiovascular mortality. Furthermore, cost–benefit analyses indicate that this form of preventative therapy is highly cost-effective.[38] If the conclusions of the recent studies are applied to all diabetic patients, then many more people with diabetes and hypertension will be alive and enjoying a better quality of life in the future.

Table 3.5 Randomized trials of antihypertensive therapy involving diabetic patients.

Trial	Patients	Number	Drugs
International Verapamil SR/Trandolapril (INVEST)	Ischaemic heart disease	27,000	Verapamil + trandolapril/atenolol hydrochlorothiazide
Losartan Intervention for End-point Reduction in hypertension (LIFE)	Left ventricular failure	9194	Losartan/atenolol
Hypertension in Veterans Trial (HYVET)	Elderly	1283	ACE/thiazide/placebo
Bergamo Nephrologic Diabetes Complications Trial (BENEDICT)	Prevention of diabetic nephropathy	2400	Verapamil + trandolapril/monotherapy
Anglo-Scandinavian Cardiac Outcomes Trial (ASCOT)	High risk	18,000	Bendrofluazide + atenolol/amlodipine + perindopril
Antihypertensive and Lipid Lowering Treatment to Prevent Heart Attack Trial (ALLHAT)	Hypertensive	40,000	Amlodipine/lisinopril/doxazosin/chlorthalidone

References

1. Dodson PM. Epidemiology and pathogenesis of hypertension in diabetes. In: AH Barnett, Dodson PM, editors. Hypertension and diabetes, 3rd edition. London: Science Press; 2000, Chapter 1.

2. Turner RC, Millns H, Neil HAW, et al. Risk factors for coronary artery disease in non-insulin dependent diabetes mellitus: United Kingdom Prospective Diabetes Study (UKPDS 23) Br Med J 1998; 316: 823–8.

3. Staessen J, Gasowki J, Wang JG, et al. Risks of untreated and treated isolated systolic hypertension in the elderly: metaanalysis of outcome trials. Lancet 2000; 355:865–72.

4. Marshall SM. Blood pressure control, microalbuminuria and cardiovascular risk in Type 2 diabetes mellitus. Diabet Med 1999; 16: 358–72.

5. Gillows JT, Gibson JM, Dodson PM. Hypertension and diabetic retinopathy – What's the story? Br J Ophthalmol 1999; 83:1083–7.

6. Curb JD, Pressel SL, Cutler JA, et al. Effect of diuretic-based antihypertensive treatment on cardiovascular disease risk in older diabetic patients with isolated systolic hypertension. Systolic Hypertension in the Elderly Program Cooperative Research Group. J Am Med Ass 1996; 276:1886–92.

7. Ramsay L, Williams B, Johnston G, et al. Guidelines for management of hypertension: report of the third working party of the British Hypertension Society. J Human Hypertens 1999, 13:569–92.

8. Anon. Joint British recommendations on prevention of coronary heart disease in clinical practice. British Cardiac Society, British Hyperlipidaemia Association, British Hypertension Society, endorsed by the British Diabetic Association. Heart 1998, 80(Suppl 2):S1–S29.

9. Vora JP, Ibrahim HAA, Bakris GL. Responding to the challenge of diabetic nephropathy: the historic evolution of detective prevention and management. J Human Hypertens 2000; 14:667–85.

10. Chowdhury TA, Kumar S, Barnett AH, Dodson PM. Treatment of hypertension in patients with type 2 diabetes: a review of the recent evidence. J Human Hypertens 1999; 13:803–11.

11. Lewis EJ, Hunsicker LG, Bain RP, et al. The effect of angiotensin-converting enzyme inhibition on diabetic nephropathy. The Collaborative Study Group. New Engl J Med 1993; 329:1456–62.

12. Lewis JB, Berl T, Bain RP, et al. Effects of intensive blood pressure control on the course of Type 1 diabetic nephropathy. Collaborative Study Group. Am J Kidney Dis 1999; 34:809–17.

13. Agardh CD, Gercia-Puig J, Charbonnel B, et al. Greater reduction of urinary albumin excretion in hypertensive Type II diabetic patients with incipient nephropathy by lisinopril than by nifendipine. J Human Hypertens 1996; 10: 185–92.

14. The EUCLID Study Group. Randomised placebo-controlled trial of lisinopril in normotensive patients with insulin-dependent diabetes and normoalbuminuria or microalbuminuria. Lancet 1997; 349: 1787–92.

15. The ACE Inhibitors in Diabetic Nephropathy Trialist Group. Should all patients with Type I diabetes mellitus and microalbuminuria receive angiotensin-converting enzyme inhibitors? Ann Intern Med 2001; 134:370–9.

16. Uager T, Azizi M, Belz GG. Blocking the tissue renin–angiotensin system: the future cornerstone of therapy. J Hum Hypertens 2000; 14(Suppl 2):S23–31.

17. Francis GS. ACE – inhibition in cardiovascular disease. Lancet 2000; 342:201–2.

18. Mogensen CE, Neldam S, Tikkanen I, et al. Randomised controlled trial of dual blockade of renin–angiotensin system in patients with hypertension, microalbuminuria, and non-insulin dependent diabetes: the candesartan and lisinopril microalbuminuria (CALM) study. Br Med J 2000; 321:1440–4.

19. Chaturvedi N, Sjolie AK, Stephenson JM, et al. Effect of lisinopril on progression of retinopathy in people with Type 1 diabetes. The EUCLID Study Group. EURODIAB Controlled Trial of Lisinopril in Insulin-Dependent Diabetes Mellitus. Lancet 1998; 351:28–31.

20. Anon. Tight blood pressure control and risk of macrovascular complications in Type 2 diabetes: UKPDS 38. UK Prospective Diabetes Study Group. Br Med J 1998; 317:703–13.

21. Hansson L, Zanchetti A, Carruthers SG, et al. Effects of intensive blood-pressure lowering and low-dose aspirin in patients with hypertension: principal results of the Hypertension Optimal Treatment (HOT) randomised trial. HOT Study Group. Lancet 1998; 351:1755–62.

22. Tuomilehto J, Rastenyte D, Birkenhäger WH, et al. Effects of calcium-channel blockade in older subjects with diabetes and systolic hypertension. Systolic hypertension in Europe trial investigators. New Engl J Med 1999; 340:677–84.

23. Anon. Effects of ramipril on cardiovascular and microvascular outcomes in people with diabetes mellitus: results of the HOPE study and MICRO-HOPE substudy. Heart Outcomes Prevention Evaluation Study Investigators. Lancet 2000; 355:253–9.

24. Hansson L, Lindgolm LH, Niskanen L, et al. Effect of angiotensin-converting enzyme inhibition compared with conventional therapy on cardiovascular morbidity and mortality in hypertension: the Captopril Prevention Project (CAPPP) randomised trial. Lancet 1999; 353: 611–16.

25. Gaede P, Vedel P, Parving HH, et al. Intensified multifactorial intervention in patients with Type 2 diabetes mellitus and micro-albuminuria: the Steno type 2 randomised study. Lancet 1999; 535:617–22.

26. Maxwell SRB, Barnett AH. The management of hypertension in the diabetic patients. In: Kendall MJ, Kaplan NM, Horton RC, editors. Difficult hypertension. London: Martin Dunitz; 1995:135–60.

27. Trost BN, Weidmann P. Effects of calcium antagonists on glucose homeostasis and serum lipids in non-diabetic and diabetic subjects: a review. J Hypertens 1987; 5(Suppl):S81–S104.

28. Estacio RO, Jeffers BW, Hiatt WR, et al. The effect of nisoldipine as compared with enalapril on cardiovascular outcomes in patients with non-insulin dependent diabetes and hypertension (ABCD Trial). New Engl J Med 1998; 338:645–52.

29. Tatti P, Pahor M, Byington RP, et al. Outcome results of the Fosinopril versus Amlodopine Cardiovascular Events Randomised Trial (FACET) in patients with hypertension and NIDDM. Diabetes Care 1998; 21(4):597–603.

30. Borhani NO, Mercuri M, Borhani PA. Final outcome results of the Multicentre Isradipine Diuretic Atherosclerosis Study (MIDAS): a randomised controlled trial. J Am Med Ass 1996; 276:785–91.

31. Anon. Efficacy of atenolol and cap-

topril in reducing risk of macrovascular and microvascular complications in type 2 diabetes: UKPDS 39. UK Prospective Diabetes Study Group. Br Med J 1998; 317:713–20.

32. McInnes GT. Angiotensin II antagonists. Br J Cardiology 1997; 4(7): 273–9.

33. Davis BR, Cutler JA, Gordon DJ, et al. Rationale and design for the Antihypertensive and Lipid Lowering treatment to Prevent Heart Attack Trial (ALLHAT). ALLHAT Research Group. Am J Hypertens 1996; 9:342–60.

34. Feher MD. Doxazosin therapy in the treatment of diabetic hypertension. Am Heart J 1991; 121:1294–301.

35. Beevers DG, Lip GYH. Do alpha blockers cause heart failure and stroke? Observations from ALLHAT. J Human Hypertens 2000; 14: 287–9.

36. Sever PS. Simple blood pressure guidelines for primary health care. J Human Hypertens 1999; 13:725–7.

37. Staessen JA, Thijs L, Fagard R, et al. Predicting cardiovascular risk using conventional vs ambulatory blood pressure in older patients with systolic hypertension. Systolic Hypertension in Europe Trial Investigators. J Am Med Ass 1999; 282:539–46.

38. Stergiou GS, Skeva II, Zoubaki AS, et al. Self-monitoring of blood pressure at home: how many measurements are needed? J Hypertens 1998; 16:725–31.

39. Anon. Cost effectiveness analysis of improved blood pressure control in hypertensive patients with type 2 diabetes: UKPDS 40. UK Prospective Diabetes Study Group. Br Med J 1998; 317:720–6.

4
How is diabetic microvascular disease best prevented and treated?

Matthew D Oldfield and Mark E Cooper

Introduction

Diabetes is the commonest endocrine disorder in the world, affecting approximately 5% of Western populations. It is significantly more prevalent in the elderly and in certain ethnic groups such as urbanized Indo-Asians. Altered population demographics, an increasingly sedentary lifestyle and the widespread adoption of Western dietary practices mean that numbers are likely to double in the next 50 years. This large disease pool implies that diabetes will continue as the leading cause of end-stage renal disease (ESRD), blindness and non-traumatic limb amputation in working-age populations in the Western world. As many as 40% of Type 1 and 10–15% of Type 2 diabetics will develop ESRD from diabetic nephropathy.[1] Substantially more diabetic subjects will manifest retinal changes after 20 years and diabetic peripheral neuropathy remains one of the most disabling long-term diabetic sequelae.

Recent interventional studies have established the benefits of strict glycaemic and blood pressure control in ameliorating the risk of microvascular complications. Further, improved understanding of the relevant pathogenic mechanisms is offering exciting new targets for future therapy.

Pathogenesis

The decades following the introduction of insulin were associated with an ominous rise in reports describing retinal and renal disease in diabetic patients. Debate regarding the relevance of glucose in the aetiology of these complications has recently been clarified with the publication of the Diabetes Control and Complications Trial (DCCT) (Figure 4.1) and the UK Prospective Diabetes Study Group (UKPDS) Group trial.[3–5] It is now established beyond reasonable doubt that glucose and blood pressure reduction is beneficial in the prevention and amelioration of microvascular disease. Genetic susceptibility and external risk factors such as

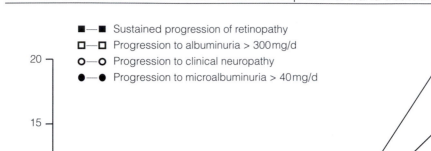

Figure 4.1

Relative risks for the development of diabetic microvascular complications at different levels of HbA1c, obtained from the Diabetes Control and Complications Trial. (Adapted from Skyler,[2] with permission.)

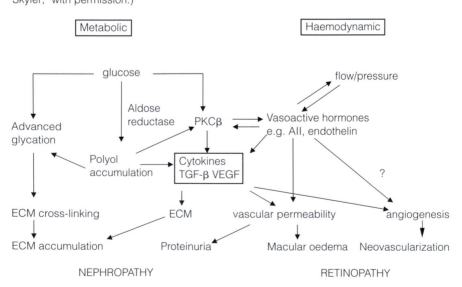

Figure 4.2

Schema for the pathogenesis of diabetic microvascular complications.

smoking have roles in modulating the complex interactions between metabolic and haemodynamic factors (Figure 4.2).

Role of hyperglycaemia

A number of equally tenable hypotheses exist for the mechanisms of hyperglycaemia-mediated microvascular damage. Traditionally considered to be separate pathways, it has recently been suggested that these metabolic alterations do not exist independently but are interlinked and stimulated collectively. In particular, the generation of reactive oxygen species by glucose may act as a common intracellular messenger system involved in the activation of several of these pathways.[6]

Metabolic alterations

Advanced glycation

Advanced glycation is a non-enzymatic post-translational modification of proteins via the spontaneous reaction of reducing sugars and the free amino groups of proteins. Early compounds, Schiff bases, undergo gradual rearrangement to form more stable ketoamines called Amadori products. Progression of the reaction occurs in proportion to the level of glycaemia. Thus, the level of Amadori products, of which glycated haemoglobin (HbA1c) is one example, is a clinically useful measure of medium-term glycaemic control. Subsequent to the generation of Amadori products, a series of condensation reactions occur that ultimately result in the formation of advanced glycation end-products (AGE).[7]

AGE formation is a ubiquitous reaction; indeed, AGE accumulate during normal ageing and may account for some physiological age-dependent vascular changes. However, AGE accumulate to a greater extent in diabetes where a substantial amount of evidence implicates that they have a pathogenic role in diabetic microvascular disease.[8]

AGE are postulated to exert their effects through two main mechanisms – direct cross-linking of proteins and binding to specific receptors. AGE-dependent covalent cross-link formation usually occurs between long-lived, stable matrix proteins such as the collagens. Modified proteins are stiffer, resistant to degradation and quench the potent vasodilator nitric oxide (NO), with detrimental effects upon tissue structure and function. The degree of AGE accumulation correlates with impairment of a number of measures of vessel function.[9]

A number of specific AGE-binding proteins have now been identified on several relevant cell types, including macrophages, smooth muscle and endothelial cells as well as on numerous cell types within the retina and kidney. Important consequences of AGE-receptor binding are the generation of soluble growth factors called cytokines as well as vaso-active hormones and procoagulants.

A number of strategies for inhibiting the process of glycation exist. Most, however, have focused upon inhibiting AGE formation using compounds such as aminoguanidine, which has repeatedly demonstrated benefits in experimental diabetes[8] and has now entered clinical trials. For example, a study termed A Clinical Trial In Overt Nephropathy (ACTION) evaluated the role of aminoguanidine as an add-on therapy in overt nephropathy.[10] Treatment with aminoguanidine in Type 1 diabetic patients with nephropathy did not statistically affect the primary end-point (a doubling of creatinine), though there were trends towards mortality reduction as well as a highly significant reduction in albuminuria and less progression of retinopathy. A number of similar agents are currently in preclinical development.

Compounds that disrupt AGE-mediated protein cross-links, such as phenacylthiazoliumbromide (PTB) and its derivative ALT 711, are exciting developments that may potentially reverse established diabetes-related tissue damage. Experimental successes in restoring vessel compliance both in non-diabetic aged[11] and in diabetic dogs[12] have now led to several clinical trials. Preliminary results from one such trial with ALT 711 noted improved measures of vessel distensability in isolated systolic hypertension,[13] a condition characterized by stiff and poorly compliant vessels.

Polyol pathway
The polyol pathway has been extensively studied in diabetic microvascular complications,[14] in particular in the pathogenesis of diabetic neuropathy. The enzyme aldose reductase catalyses the conversion of glucose to sorbitol, using reduced nicotinamide–adenine dinucleotide phosphate (NADPH) as a cofactor. In the context of hyperglycaemia, the metabolism of high levels of glucose causes sorbitol accumulation and the consumption of NADPH. Increased levels of sorbitol are associated with depletion of intracellular myoinositol, reduced sodium/potassium adenosine triphosphatase (ATPase) activity, osmotic damage and reduced nerve conduction velocities.

Consumption of NADPH changes cellular redox potential. NADPH is required for NO synthase to produce NO and in the regeneration of the free-radical scavenger glutathione. Reduced NO may contribute to neurovascular ischaemia.[15]

Although the polyol pathway and AGE formation are usually considered to be separate pathways, the subsequent metabolism of sorbitol to fructose creates a reducing sugar that enters the AGE pathway. Sorbinil, an aldose reductase inhibitor (ARI), was reported to prevent sorbitol accumulation and reduce AGE-mediated cross-linking of the extracellular matrix.[16]

These ARI have allowed investigators to explore the role of polyols in diabetic complications. These agents have shown promise in the prevention of cataract formation and in improving or stabilizing diabetic neuropathy. In the short term, ARI also blunt glomerular hyperfiltration and attenuate albuminuria.[17] However, the benefits upon diabetic nephropathy and retinopathy appear mild and clinical trials of ARI in humans have, in general, been disappointing. Their role in diabetic neuropathy will be discussed later.

Protein Kinase C (PKC) activation

A direct pathogenic role for glucose has been suggested by cell culture experiments demonstrating that glucose itself could induce cellular hypertrophy, extracellular matrix synthesis and cytokine production. These effects have been attributed to activation of protein kinase C (PKC), a ubiquitous family of serine/threonine kinases that are increased in the retina, aorta, heart and glomeruli of diabetic animals. Radiolabelling of glucose shows that glycolytic intermediates are incorporated directly into the glycerol backbone of compounds called diacylglycerol (DAG), the major endogenous activator of PKC. This results in a de novo increase in DAG and PKC activation. A second relevant pathway also exists. Ligands such as angiotensin II (Ang II), vascular endothelial growth factor (VEGF) and endothelin bind to a cell membrane G-protein coupled receptor and initiate a phospholipid cascade that also generates DAG.

The PKC family regulates a diverse range of vascular functions including blood flow regulation, cellular differentiation and cytokine generation. The observation that there is preferential activation of the β isoform of PKC in diabetes has led to the development and study of isoform-specific inhibitors such as LY 333531.[18] Significant amelioration of diabetes-dependent abnormalities of retinal blood flow and glomerular hyperfiltration have been demonstrated in experimental diabetes and the compound has now entered clinical trials, primarily in retinopathy, in the USA and Europe.

Renin–Angiotensin system (RAS)

A role for the renin–angiotensin system (RAS) is strongly suggested by clinical trials of angiotensin-converting-enzyme (ACE) inhibitors that show benefits in diabetic renal and retinal disease. It has been reported that the RAS is locally activated in the diabetic retina[19] and kidney.[20] In addition to the role Ang II plays in haemodynamics, it is also known to act as a growth factor in its own right, in part through activation of PKC. Animal studies have shown that ACE inhibitors reduce PKC activation[21] and ameliorate both diabetes-dependent increases in retinal VEGF[22] and renal transforming growth factor β (TGF-β).[23]

Cytokines

An area of intense research interest has focused on the properties of soluble growth factors called cytokines. Overexpression and inappropriate expression of these powerful molecules is believed to play a central role in the development of microvascular disease.

TGF-β is thought to be the pivotal cytokine involved in a number of fibrotic conditions including diabetic nephropathy.[24] TGF-β coordinates the physiological process of normal tissue repair, potently stimulating matrix protein production and inhibiting its degradation. In addition, TGF-β has a number of powerful effects upon cellular differentiation and proliferation. Overexpression of TGF-β in gene-tranfection experiments caused the development of glomerulosclerosis and fibrosis. Administration of TGF-β neutralizing antibodies, in a mouse model of Type 2 diabetes, prevented the observed diabetes-dependent accumulation of glomerular matrix and the development of tubulointerstitial fibrosis.[25] TGF-β neutralization also prevented the diabetes-related decrease in glomerular filtration rate, though interestingly it failed to normalize proteinuria. This indicates that one cannot assume that albuminuria and renal structural changes will behave in a similar manner to various renoprotective therapies.

The theory of the pathogenesis of diabetic retinopathy has focused upon the existence of diffusible angiogenic factors present in the retina and stimulated by hypoxia. The glycoprotein VEGF appears to satisfy the criteria as a major mediator of diabetic retinopathy.[26] It is present in a number of cells in the retina, including pericytes, Müller cells and retinal pigment epithelial cells and is upregulated up to 15-fold by hypoxia. In addition, activation of PKC by hyperglycaemia and Ang II also increases VEGF expression.

VEGF has a number of roles in physiological angiogenesis and its ability to potently increase vascular permeability makes it an attractive candidate for playing a role in the development of macular oedema. VEGF levels in intraocular fluid from diabetic subjects undergoing surgery correlate with the presence of active neovascular disease and the levels reduce when retinal disease becomes quiescent.[27] Other supportive data comes from models of ischaemic retinopathy, where the administration of VEGF inhibitors was shown to prevent neovascularization.[26]

Compared to the kidney and retina, much less is known about the role of growth factors in the pathogenesis of diabetic neuropathy. The target organs of sympathetic and parasympathetic innervation produce neurotrophic growth factors such as nerve growth factor (NGF). The retrograde transport of these to the neuronal cell body is a requirement for normal nerve growth and maintenance. Loss of neurotrophic support, theoretically at least, would render neurons less resistant to injury.

Insulin-like growth factor (IGF)-1 has also been implicated in maintaining normal nerve differentiation and plasticity.

A number of other cytokines have also been implicated in the development of microvascular complications and it appears that a complex interplay among growth factors takes place. One important feature is that upregulation of these cytokines occurs with both the metabolic and haemodynamic alterations occurring in diabetes (Figure 4.2). This activation of cytokines may represent a common pathway, one that offers an attractive target for disease modification.

Diabetic retinopathy

Diabetic retinopathy is a well-characterized, potentially sight-threatening complication that eventually develops to some degree in nearly all diabetic subjects. Experienced ophthalmological evaluation can detect diabetic retinopathy in its early stages. Effective treatments exist but require appropriate and timely implementation, thus preventative measures remain a cornerstone of management.

Clinical and natural histories

Diabetic retinopathy generally progresses through well-characterized stages, associated with typical pathological changes. Before the onset of detectable disease there are alterations in retinal blood flow, loss of retinal pericytes and thickening of basement membranes. The development of vascular microaneurysms and blot haemorrhages constitute background disease, and is associated with compromised barrier function. Increased vascular permeability allows exudation of lipoproteins, seen as hard exudates. With disease progression, the gradual loss of the retinal circulation results in areas of ischaemia. Venous calibre alterations (beading), intra-retinal microvascular abnormalities (IRMA), extensive localized haemorrhages and microaneurysm formation are commonly seen at this stage. In proliferative disease, friable new vessel formation in the retina and iris occurs as a consequence of ischaemic stimuli. These vessels are prone to spontaneous bleeding and, in later stages, may undergo fibrosis and contraction, with subsequent retinal detachment. Areas of oedema may develop and, if sufficiently close to the fovea, may threaten sight. Irreversible vision loss can occur through a number of mechanisms such as macular oedema, and new vessels may bleed or produce tractional retinal detachment; ultimately, neovascular glaucoma may develop.

Pathogenesis

The hypoxia theory of retinal neovascularization was proposed 50 years ago by Michaelson.[28] Work in other ischaemic retinopathies has implicated VEGF as a major mediator, as noted earlier.[27]

A number of other growth factors are also likely to play a role in neovascularization. Levels of IGF-1 correlate with the deterioration in retinopathy sometimes seen following improvements in glycaemic control. Roles for oestrogen and basic fibroblast growth factor (bFGF) have also been described.[27] bFGF initiates endothelial mitosis and is released from cells under hypoxic conditions, potentially playing an important permissive role with VEGF in neovascularization.

Glycaemia and blood pressure

A number of epidemiological studies have described the relationship between diabetes and the onset and progression of diabetic retinopathy. For example, the Wisconsin Epidemiological Study of Diabetic Retinopathy (WESDR) identified 1200 patients with younger onset and 1800 with late-onset diabetes, and described the relationship between the onset of retinopathy and the duration of diabetes. In addition, this study established that progression of retinopathy was a function of baseline disease, i.e. the more severe the disease the greater the frequency of progression to sight-threatening pathology. This has formed the basis for initial screening recommendations.

The importance of glucose control has been confirmed by trials such as the DCCT,[3] where intensive insulin treatment reduced or prevented the development of retinopathy by 27% compared to conventional therapy. In addition, intensive treatment caused a 76% reduction in sustained three-step or greater progression on the Early Treatment Diabetic Retinopathy Study (ETDRS) research group scale. The risk of neovascularization was also significantly reduced.

The UKPDS data demonstrated that glycaemia at baseline and glycaemic exposure through the course of the study were related to the risk of developing new disease, and also to the risk of progression of established retinopathy in Type 2 diabetes.[29] Intensive blood glucose control significantly reduced the risk of retinopathy development compared to conventional control. All microvascular complications were reduced by approximately 35% for every 1% reduction in HbA1c.[4]

It is important to note that in both trials even patients receiving intensive treatment had some progression of their disease. In the DCCT study it took 3 years before a clear difference between intensive and conventional treatment was observed, suggesting that targeting of other risk factors is also required. The detrimental effect of blood pressure has been seen in a number of trials in diabetes, including the UKPDS. Analysis of the sorbinil retinopathy trial, a cohort of 485 Type 1 diabetic subjects identified prospectively, demonstrated that the progression of retinal disease was related to diastolic blood pressure; this finding is consistent with work from other trials.[30] The UKPDS demonstrated an association between blood pressure and the development of new retinal disease. The risk of new disease was reduced by 34% in the group assigned to tight blood pressure control.

Choice of antihypertensive agent

The recognition of Ang II-mediated growth effects and the correlation of pro-renin, ACE and Ang II levels to disease severity have focused attention upon agents that modulate the RAS. The Eurodiab Controlled Trial of Lisinopril in Insulin-dependent Diabetes (EUCLID) trial[31] studied Type 1 diabetic subjects who were predominantly normoalbuminuric and normotensive. Of the cohort, 65% had evidence of retinopathy at baseline. Treatment with lisinopril reduced the risk of a one-stage ETDRS deterioration by 50%. The risk of a two-stage deterioration was also reduced significantly over the 2 years of the study. In addition, there was a non-significant risk reduction (30%) for the development of new disease. Benefits were independent of baseline retinopathy and, despite a 3mmHg difference between groups, adjustments for blood pressure differences suggested that systemic blood pressure differences did not fully account for the benefit in those receiving lisinopril.

The UKPDS trial demonstrated no differences in outcome benefit between groups treated with captopril and atenolol. However, this study cannot be considered a direct comparison since most patients in the study were on two or more drugs.[32]

Treatment of established disease

Retinal photocoagulation

Retinal photocoagulation is the only treatment modality with a documented effect upon established diabetic retinopathy.[33] The primary therapy for proliferative diabetic retinopathy (PDR) is pan-retinal photocoagulation, which, if applied in an appropriate and timely manner, can prevent 95% of visual loss resulting from PDR. Cryotherapy or vitrectomy with endophotocoagulation may be tried when laser photocoagulation is not possible.

Beneficial effects are assumed to result from the reduction of retinal ischaemic load through destruction of ischaemic retina, with a reduction in growth factor release. Whilst dramatically effective treatment is a significant event in a patient's life, photocoagulation causes some discomfort and reduces both peripheral and night vision. Focal photocoagulation for the treatment of macular oedema is less effective, although 50% of moderate visual loss may be preventable with this form of treatment.

Intraocular surgery can drain vitreal haemorrhages, divide fibrous bands and reattach detached areas of retina.

Screening
The irreversible and frequently silent development of retinal changes in diabetes means that early detection is vitally important. The risk of progression to sight-threatening disease is proportional to the current retinal stage. In Type1 diabetes, retinopathy is unlikely to develop within 5 years of diagnosis; therefore, it is recommended that Type 1 diabetic subjects should be examined within 3–5 years of diagnosis. A significant proportion (37%) of Type 2 patients in the UKPDS trial had established retinopathy at entry, reflecting the longer disease duration prediagnosis. Screening should therefore start immediately after diagnosis in Type 2 diabetic subjects. The frequency of follow-up depends upon the disease stage observed at the initial screening.

Future therapies
More detailed understanding of the role cytokines play in the pathogenesis of retinopathy has suggested new treatment targets. Locally injected VEGF inhibitors have dramatically ameliorated experimental neovascularization.[34] In addition, upstream and downstream targeting of intracellular signaling pathways, e.g. inhibiting PKC activation, has led to reductions of retinal VEGF expression.[26]

Angiostatin, a novel angiogenesis inhibitor has recently been reported to potently inhibit endothelial proliferation in vitro, possibly through bFGF-dependent mechanisms.

Thalidomide is a well-known potent teratogen. It is postulated that its teratogenicity may relate to an ability to inhibit blood vessel growth in the developing fetal limb bud. A study of the effects of thalidomide on growing vasculature on the rabbit cornea and chicken chorioallantoic membrane showed that thalidomide is an inhibitor of bFGF-induced angiogenesis.

Further studies should ascertain whether these two compounds have a useful role in the treatment and prevention of diabetic retinopathy.

Special circumstances
PDR, regardless of the duration of diabetes, is rare in children before puberty; however, puberty may accelerate the progression of retinopathy. Similarly, pregnancy can cause a more aggressive progression of diabetic retinopathy. Thus, pregnant diabetic women should have a comprehensive eye examination within 1 year of conception and close follow-up throughout pregnancy is recommended. This does not apply to patients with gestational diabetes, as they are not at risk of PDR.

Diabetic nephropathy (DN)

Natural history

With the onset of hyperglycaemia, structural and haemodynamic changes are quickly detectable in the kidney. The earliest changes include an increase in the glomerular filtration rate (GFR) of up to 150%. This increase is paralleled by an increase in renal size, resulting primarily from renal hypertrophy but also from an increase in cell proliferation. The next observable change is the development of increased rates of urinary albumin excretion of 30–300mg/day (microalbuminuria). Special assay techniques are required, as this level is below the detection level of conventional urinary dipsticks. Persistent microalbuminuria is associated with changes both in glomerular structure (mesangial matrix expansion and basement membrane thickening) and permeability, and is sometimes referred to as incipient nephropathy. These changes occur in 30–50% of Type 1 diabetic subjects 5–10 years after the onset of diabetes, but may be present in 20–30% of Type 2 diabetic subjects at the time of initial diagnosis.

The development of persistent microalbuminuria is associated with a markedly increased risk of developing macroproteinuria and in the progression to end-stage renal failure. The majority (80%) of Type 1 patients who develop microalbuminuria within the first 10 years will progress to frank diabetic nephropathy (DN). A lower percentage (20–40%) of Type 2 diabetic subjects with microalbuminuria will progress to nephrotic range proteinuria within 10 years. Histologically, glomeruli show glomerular basement membrane (GBM) thickening and mesangial expansion, eventually resulting in diffuse and/or focal nodular glomerulosclerosis, afferent and efferent arteriolar sclerosis, and tubulointerstitial fibrosis.

Haemodynamics

It has been suggested that the earliest predictor for the development of DN is hyperfiltration. This is especially so in Type 1 diabetes, where a GFR > 125ml/min carries a 50% risk compared with 5% in those with a GFR < 125ml/min of the development of microalbuminuria over an 8-year time period. However, this concept for a predictive role for hyperfiltration is not a universal finding. The mechanisms involved in increasing GFR involve glucose-dependent effects on arteriolar dilatation, mediated by a range of vasoactive factors including Ang II, IGF-1, NO and prostaglandins.

Experimentally, this hyperfiltration is mediated by afferent arteriolar dilatation with an increase in glomerular hydrostatic pressure. Measures that reduce glomerular pressure, such as systemic blood pressure reduction, a low-protein diet or ACE inhibitors that block Ang II-mediated efferent arteriolar constriction, all reduce the development of glomerular damage and proteinuria.

Pathogenesis

Familial clustering of DN suggests a possible genetic basis for this complication, though no gene has been clearly shown to determine DN susceptibility.[35] Some studies have proposed a link between DN and the double-deletion ACE genotype. However, not all studies have shown a significant association.[36]

The mechanisms linking chronic hyperglycaemia and hypertension to the development of DN have recently begun to be unravelled. It was recognized at the Joslin Clinic soon after the introduction of insulin that poor glycaemic control and disease duration were risk factors for the development of DN; this has now been firmly established by the findings from the DCCT and UKPDS. With good glycaemic control only 9% of Type 1 diabetic subjects will develop ESRD after 25 years, compared to a historical prevalence of 40%.[37]

Numerous studies have shown that control of systemic hypertension has a major effect on reducing proteinuria and slowing progression to renal failure in both Type 1 and Type 2 diabetes.[38]

Prevention and treatment

Glycaemic control
Normoalbuminuria to microalbuminuria
The importance of strict glycaemic control was best shown by the DCCT. Type 1 subjects randomized to receive tight glycaemic control had a 35-45% lower risk for the development of microalbuminuria than those receiving conventional therapy.[3]

In the UKPDS trial, Type 2 diabetic subjects randomized to receive intensive glycaemic treatment had a HbA1c on average 0.9% lower than those treated conventionally. This was associated with a 25–30% reduction for the development of microalbuminuria and proteinuria, and > 50% reduction in the number of patients with a doubling of serum creatinine.[4] In the Kumamoto study of 110 Japanese non-obese and young (mean age 50 years) Type 2 diabetic subjects, intensive insulin treatment reduced the risk of developing microalbuminuria by 62% and albuminuria by 100% in the primary prevention cohort. In a secondary prevention group, defined as the presence of retinopathy, intensive treatment caused a risk reduction for microalbuminuria of 52% and macroalbuminuria of 100%. In that study, a HbA1c threshold existed at 6.5%, below which the risk for the development of microalbuminuria was negligible.[39]

Progression of microalbuminuria and macroproteinuria

The evidence that intensive glycaemic control slows the progression of DN, once microalbuminuria is persistent, is more controversial. Within the DCCT few patients had established microalbuminuria at entry, and although in the intensive treatment group fewer patients progressed to frank albuminuria this did not reach statistical significance. A similar non-significant trend was shown in the Microalbuminuria Collaborative Study Group from the UK. However, several Scandinavian studies have reported slower progression to DN in microalbuminuric subjects receiving intensive glucose control. Similarly, a study from Guys Hospital, London, reported that intensive glucose control prevented progression if blood pressure was well controlled. The frequent occurrence of hypertension in DN may represent a powerful confounding factor explaining the failure of some of the reported studies to reach statistical significance.

Antihypertensive therapy

It is clear that hypertension, or a rise in blood pressure within the normal range, is common in the early stages of DN and is partly related to sodium retention and volume expansion. The association between hypertension and DN was first described by Kimmelstiel and Wilson in 1936,[40] though the adverse effect of hypertension in diabetic (and non-diabetic) renal disease was not appreciated until later. In the UKPDS trial, tight blood pressure control was associated with a 37% reduction in microvascular end-points [95% confidence interval (CI) 11–56%]; a number of other studies show concordance with this finding. In established DN studies, by Parving and others, it has been demonstrated that blood pressure control decreases albuminuria and reduces the rate of GFR decline from approximately 10 to < 5ml/year.[38]

A major question relates to what level of blood pressure constitutes hypertension in diabetic patients. The modification of Diet in Renal Disease Study of non-diabetic patients with renal disease provided strong evidence that achieving a lower blood pressure (125/75mmHg) was associated with a slower rate of progression in patients with proteinuria compared with standard blood pressure goals (140/90mmHg). These observations, as well as others, led the Sixth Joint National Committee to recommend the more aggressive antihypertensive target of 125/75mmHg in proteinuric diabetic patients, with commencement of treatment at 130/85mmHg.[41]

Are ACE inhibitors better than other agents?

A second and much-debated area relates to the type of antihypertensive therapy used. In particular, do ACE inhibitors confer additional treatment benefits over more conventional agents?

Whilst a number of studies have clearly documented that ACE inhibitors will reduce proteinuria of any etiology by 40–50%, and retard the development of frank proteinuria, it has been difficult to separate the effects of ACE inhibition from blood pressure reduction. Most studies have compared ACE inhibition with placebo; consequently, blood pressure differences usually exist between the groups. Two recent meta-analyses, that included both short- and long-term-treated patients with micro- and macroalbuminuria, have demonstrated an enhanced antiproteinuric benefit attributed to the use of ACE inhibitors over β-blockers and diuretics, independent of blood pressure reduction.[42,43]

Primary prevention

An unresolved issue is whether the benefits observed in microalbuminuric patients can be extended to diabetic patients prior to the onset of microalbuminuria. At the end of the EUCLID study the albumin excretion rate (AER) was reduced by 19% (an absolute difference of 2.2μg/min) by the ACE inhibitor lisinopril, in a predominantly normoalbuminuric and normotensive population.[31] The significance of such a reduction is not yet clear, interestingly, it appears that the risk of progression to microalbuminuria, at least in Type 1 diabetic subjects, is highest in those with AER in the upper limit of the normal range.

This issue has not been extensively studied in Type 2 diabetes, in part because most Type 2 diabetic subjects are hypertensive at presentation.

Micro- and macroalbuminuria and normotension
A recent meta-analysis by the ACE inhibitors in Diabetic Nephropathy Trialists Group considered a number of placebo-controlled trials of ACE inhibitors in microalbuminuric and normotensive Type 1 diabetic subjects (Figure 4.3). ACE inhibitors significantly reduced the progression of micro- to macroalbuminuria and increased the chances of regression to normoalbuminuria.[44] The authors concluded that blood pressure changes could not entirely explain the antiproteinuric benefit of ACE inhibitors. In a group of predominantly Type 1 diabetic normotensive subjects with microalbuminuria, Marre[45] reported that enalapril treatment for 12 months retarded the development of macroalbuminuria. Similar results could not be achieved using equally hypotensive doses of a thiazide diuretic, suggesting superior benefits with ACE inhibition.[46]

The Melbourne Diabetic Nephropathy study group compared nifedipine and perindopril in Type 1 normotensive, microalbuminuric patients. In the dihydropyridine group there was both an increase in AER and a decline in GFR compared to the group receiving the ACE inhibitor.[47,48] However, in a similar comparison, Crepaldi et al.[49] compared lisinopril and nifedipine, demonstrating a reduction in AER for both groups (significantly more with the ACE inhibitor). Despite the quantitative difference in AER reduction, no differences were seen in the rate of GFR decline over 3 years.

A number of studies exist in normotensive Type 2 diabetic subjects. Ravid et al.[50] demonstrated long-term stabilization of plasma creatinine levels and a reduced risk of developing proteinuria in enalapril-treated Type 2 diabetic subjects.[50,51] Sano et al.[52] compared 28 patients treated with enalapril to placebo-treated controls in a similar population. Enalapril lowered urinary albumin excretion but there was no change in renal function as assessed by creatinine clearance in either group.

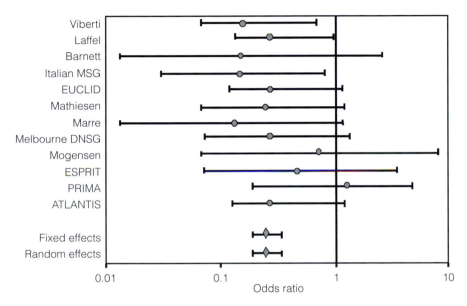

Figure 4.3

Meta-analysis of the effects of ACE inhibitors upon the risk of progression from micro- to macroalbuminuria in normotensive Type 1 diabetic patients. From the ACE inhibitors in Diabetic Nephropathy Trialist Group,[44] with permission.

Microalbuminuric/proteinuric patients with hypertension

Most studies have shown that ACE inhibitors can reduce proteinuria of any etiology by 40–50%. However, there is evidence that, in addition to reducing proteinuria, ACE inhibitors slow the deterioration of renal function. In the Collaborative Study Group Trial, captopril treatment was compared to placebo in Type 1 diabetic subjects with proteinuria (> 500mg/day) and mildly impaired renal function (mean serum creatinine > 115μmol/l). Treatment was associated with a slowing of the decline of renal function over the 3-year study period (11 versus 17% decline in creatinine clearance per year).[53] Remission of nephrotic levels of proteinuria occurred in seven of 42 individuals taking captopril but in only one of 66 controls.[54]

In a 45-month study in established DN, the Steno group demonstrated equivalent protection of GFR by captopril and nisoldipine for an equal reduction of blood pressure. This was despite an increase in proteinuria in the nisoldipine group.

In Type 2 diabetes, ACE inhibitors have also been shown to be more potent at reducing proteinuria than conventional therapy. It is less evident whether ACE inhibitors are superior to other antihypertensive medications in Type 2 diabetic subjects with albuminuria. In general, most studies have shown some advantage to either ACE inhibitors or non-dihydropyridine calcium-channel blockers when compared with the dihydropyridines, both in reducing proteinuria and stabilizing renal function.

In the UKPDS trial, significant renal protection was achieved in new or early disease, regardless of the agent used (atenolol or captopril), although this did not represent a direct comparison of the two treatments.

Two large studies in macroproteinuric Type 2 diabetic subjects using ATI receptor blockers have now been reported.[55,56] These studies indicate that ATI receptor blockers confer superior renoprotection than agents which do not interrupt the RAS including calcium channel blockers. Furthermore, in the recently reported IRMA 2 study,[57] the AII antagonist, irbesartan, was shown to retard the development of overt proteinuria in hypertensive, microalbuminuric Type 2 diabetic subjects in a dose dependent manner.

Dietary protein intake and lipotoxicity

Several small studies have suggested that dietary protein restriction may slow the progressive loss of renal function in DN, and the American Diabetes Association (ADA) now recommends that non-pregnant diabetic patients should restrict their daily protein intake to 0.8g/kg ideal body weight.

It has also been suggested that lipid-lowering therapy may confer renoprotective benefits to diabetic patients. There are a number of theoretical reasons why lipids could accelerate renal injury, including activation of cytokine-dependent pathways and stimulation of macrophage proliferation and recruitment.[58] A number of small studies have suggested that HMG CoA reductase inhibitors may confer renoprotection and reduce proteinuria, although this has not been a universal finding.[59,60]

Management

Microalbuminuria represents an ideal stage for intervention, as no established loss of renal function has developed. Improved metabolic control and antihypertensive therapies stabilize, or even reduce, microalbuminuria, as well as slowing the progression to established renal disease. The method of blood pressure reduction may be less important than the achievement of target blood pressure, which may require multiple agents.

Diabetic neuropathy

Diabetic neuropathy is one of the most frequent complications of diabetes and accounts for more hospital admissions than all the other complications combined. Diabetic neuropathy is not a distinct entity and consists of a number of clinical syndromes that affect characteristic regions of the nervous system, either singly or in combination. It is typified by a progressive loss of nerve fibres and this can be assessed in a variety of ways including clinical sensory and detailed quantitative neuronal and autonomic testing and electrophysiology.

Classification

Numerous classification schemes for diabetic neuropathy have been proposed and are usually based upon clinical presentation. A popular and widely accepted anatomical classification is that of Thomas.[61]

Pathogenesis

The pathogenesis of diabetic neuropathy remains poorly understood, but it is likely to be multifactorial. In common with other microvascular complications, neuropathy shares a relation to diabetes duration and control; however, differences in the pathogenesis of neuropathy are believed to exist. A great deal of research has focused upon metabolic consequences of diabetes, in particular the role of the polyol pathway and the consequences of sorbitol accumulation. A study by Tomlinson et al.[15] showed that, despite restoring nerve conduction velocity (NCV), ARI did not restore normal doppler flow; it remains unclear to what extent nerve dysfunction in diabetes is a result of metabolic or vascular alterations.

One of the earliest studies to establish a relationship between glucose control and neuropathy was performed by Pirart,[62] who assessed neuropathy clinically and measured glucose, both on an annual basis. Poor control was associated with a higher incidence of neuropathy.

Glycaemic control

Intensive glucose control in the DCCT study decreased the incidence of diabetic neuropathy to 3%, compared to 10% in the group that received conventional treatment. The risk of progression from subclinical to overt neuropathy was also reduced from 16 to 7% by intensive treatment. This effect was significant for clinical examination and clinical testing, though marginal for autonomic testing.

Meticulous glycaemic control through use of a continuous insulin infusion in the Oslo study resulted in significantly improved motor conduction velocities and sensory action potential amplitudes.[63] In another small and short-term study, insulin infusion improved autonomic nerve function. Trials in Type 2 diabetic subjects have been less numerous but the UKPDS trial demonstrated a reduced risk for the development of neuropathy.

Transplantation of pancreatic tissue in animals with experimental diabetic neuropathy has successfully restored NCV to normal; however, the benefits in humans are less certain. Solders et al[64] followed patients for 2 years after a combined kidney–pancreatic transplant and compared these subjects to those receiving only a kidney transplant. There was no difference in either somatic or autonomic function over the short study duration. A 10-year long-term study demonstrated some modest improvements in motor nerve conduction velocities. In addition, in some cases a small improvement in clinical measures of nerve function was observed in those receiving a pancreas compared to those awaiting transplantation.[65] Evidence for benefits in neuropathy have primarily focused upon polyneuropathy. Amyotrophy and single or multiple mononeuropathies have been specifically excluded in studies of improved glycaemic control.

ACE inhibition

The UKPDS trial demonstrated a significant reduction in all microvascular complications with tighter blood pressure control. ACE inhibitors are now established in offering benefits in the development and progression of diabetic kidney and retinal disease. Interestingly, a recent study by Malik[66] suggested that the ACE inhibitor quinapril improved measures of autonomic neuropathy. In a 12-month study of trandolapril treatment significant improvements in peripheral nerve function were observed. This role of ACE inhibitors as neuro-protective agents remains to be clearly delineated.

Aldose reductase inhibition

ARI have been around for many years and reduce the conversion of glucose to sorbitol. They have been extensively studied in experimental models of diabetic neuropathy. Use of the ARI sorbinil demonstrated significant benefits in neuropathy, preventing the diabetes-related decline in NCV in diabetic dogs over a 5-year study period.[67] However, clinical trials have been disappointing. A recent meta-analysis by Nicolucci et al[68] of randomized control trials involving ARI demonstrated a modest benefit of treatment in only one aspect – improved median nerve motor conduction velocity. The majority of trials failed to reach statistical significance on their own and a lack of hard end-point benefits, coupled with intra-trial heterogeneity, has rendered the evidence for the use of ARI in humans as unconvincing.

Newer treatments

Alpha lipoic acid (ALA) and gamma linolenic acid (GLA)

ALA acts as a cofactor in the pyruvate dehydrogenase complex and is believed to act as a redox-modulating agent. In smaller, short-term trials ALA has demonstrated significant improvements in nerve conduction studies and is undergoing clinical trials in the USA.[69]

The essential fatty acid linoleic acid is metabolized to GLA, which serves as an important membrane constituent and as a substrate for the generation of prostaglandin E formation. In diabetes this conversion to GLA is impaired and may contribute to diabetic neuropathy. A recent 1-year, multicentre trial of GLA administration to patients with diabetic neuropathy reported improved clinical and electrophysiological measures of nerve function.[70]

Novel treatments

The administration of recombinant NGF (rNGF) in a prospective, placebo-controlled phase II trial demonstrated significant improvements in a range of neurological end-points, including cold detection and vibration perception thresholds. The follow-on phase III trial comprised over 1000 patients but was unable to confirm these encouraging findings, therefore the role of rNGF remains uncertain.[71]

Symptomatic treatment

Pain control

One of the most difficult management issues in diabetic neuropathy is pain control. There is no single therapy that will benefit all patients with painful diabetic neuropathy. Management follows a stepwise approach from the use of simple analgesics to more complex agents.

Antidepressants

The analgesic effect of tricylic antidepressants appears to be independent of their antidepressant mode of action and occurs more rapidly. A meta-analysis of 21 different trials, including tricyclics, demonstrated significant pain relief in 30% of patients with neuropathic pain.[72] Amitriptyline, imipramine, clomipramine and nortriptyline have all been shown to be more effective than placebo, allowing the selection of individual agents with comparatively advantageous side-effect profiles.

The selective serotonin reuptake inhibitors (SSRI) paroxetine and citalopram have also been reported to be more effective than placebo in reducing pain, though less so than imipramine. Venlafaxine, a serotonin and noradrenaline reuptake inhibitor, also has reported beneficial effects.[73] Mianserin was not shown to be effective in one randomized controlled trial.

Anticonvulsants
Only four randomized clinical trials of the agents phenytoin, carbamazepine and gabapentin exist.[74] Carbamazepine has been reported to confer benefit in a single, double-blind crossover-trial that included a variety of diabetic neuropathic syndromes. In a large multicentre randomized controlled trial, involving both Type 1 and Type 2 diabetic patients, gabapentin significantly decreased pain scores and improved quality of life[75]; the maximum dose used was higher than that recommended for epilepsy therapy. However, as benefits were seen during the drug titration phase, the use of lower doses may offer benefits with a reduced risk of side effects. Studies of phenytoin have produced conflicting results.

Capsaicin
Marked hyperaesthesia with burning is typical of C-fibre pain which may respond to capsaicin, a topical application derived from chilli pepper. Chronic administration depletes the neurotransmitter substance P. A number of trials have demonstrated the effectiveness of capsaicin in treating neuropathic pain, though this has not been a universal finding.[76] In a comparative study comparing capsaicin and amitryptiline there was little difference in efficacy.[77] However, it should be appreciated that studies with capsaicin are difficult to effectively blind.

Clonidine
Sympathetic blocking agents such as clonidine can lessen the pain derived from sympathetically mediated C fibres in a subset of patients.

Local analgesics
Slow intravenous infusion of lignocaine was beneficial in one double-blind cross-over study and in two uncontrolled studies.[78] Mexiletine, an oral analogue, relieved painful neuropathic symptoms in a longer cross-over study.[79] Benefits are believed to occur through the stabilization of excitable neurons.

Autonomic neuropathy

Abnormalities in well-established cardiac risk factors cannot entirely explain the excessive cardiovascular mortality in diabetic subjects. The development of autonomic neuropathy is a significant cardiac risk factor and is associated with an increased risk of sudden death. Strict control of glucose, lipids and blood pressure and the use of ACE inhibitors have all been shown to reduce the odds ratio for the development of autonomic neuropathy. A number of specific treatments offer benefits to selected individuals, some of which are discussed below.

The management of postural hypotension presents a difficult problem, as augmenting standing blood pressure may have detrimental effects upon the cardiovascular blood pressure load. Supportive garments remain a first-line therapy, though a number of patients benefit from flu-drocortisone and supplementary salt intake. Unfortunately, the therapeutic window is small and symptoms often do not improve until oedema develops.

Multiple small feeds are the first step in managing diabetic gastroparesis. Reducing the amount of dietary fat may also improve gastric emptying. Pharmacological therapies include dopamine antagonism with metoclopramide and domperidone, and the motilin agonist erythromycin. Ultimately, jejunostomy placement may need to be considered.

Erectile dysfunction occurs in 50–75% of diabetic men. The multifactorial aetiology requires not only an accurate assessment of drug intake, autonomic function and vascular status but also a careful consideration of the patient's psychogenic status. Sildenafil is effective in < 50% of diabetic patients and higher doses are often required than those for the general population. The interaction with nitrates currently restricts the use of this compound in patients with underlying cardiovascular disease and may thus disqualify many diabetic patients. Transurethral applications of alprostadil, or intrapenile injections of papaverine and regitine, have been reported to provide satisfactory sexual function in 60–87% of patients, but are less acceptable to them.

Conclusions

Recent trials have demonstrated that prevention of new disease and amelioration of established pathology can be achieved through aggressive glucose and blood pressure management. Despite this evidence, diabetic patients are often undertreated and the attainment of current treatment goals in the everyday population remains a major challenge. Improved understanding of the metabolic and haemodynamic pathways involved in diabetes has identified specific treatment targets, and offers hope for the future treatment and prevention of microvascular complications.

References

1. Cooper ME. Pathogenesis, prevention, and treatment of diabetic nephropathy. Lancet 1998; 352: 213–19.

2. Skyler JS. Diabetic complications. The importance of glucose control. Endocr Metab Clin North Am 1996; 25:243–54.

3. The Diabetes Control and Complications Trial Research Group. The effect of intensive treatment of diabetes on the development and progression of long-term complications in insulin-dependent diabetes mellitus. New Engl J Med 1993; 329:977–86.

4. UK Prospective Diabetes Study (UKPDS) Group. Intensive blood-glucose control with sulphonylureas or insulin compared with conventional treatment and risk of complications in patients with type 2 diabetes (UKPDS 33). Lancet 1998; 352:837–53.

5. UK Prospective Diabetes Study (UKPDS) Group. Effect of intensive blood-glucose control with metformin on complications in overweight patients with type 2 diabetes (UKPDS 34). Lancet 1998; 352:854–65.

6. Nishikawa T, Edelstein D, Brownlee M. The missing link: a single unifying mechanism for diabetic complications. Kidney Int 2000; 58(Suppl 77): S26–S30.

7. Bucala R, Vlassara H. Advanced glycosylation end products in diabetic renal and vascular disease. Am J Kidney Dis 1995; 26:875–88.

8. Soulis-Liparota T, Cooper M, Papazoglou D, et al. Retardation by aminoguanidine of development of albuminuria, mesangial expansion, and tissue fluorescence in streptozocin-induced diabetic rat. Diabetes 1991; 40: 1328–34.

9. Airaksinen KE, Salmela PI, Linnaluoto MK, et al. Diminished arterial elasticity in diabetes: association with fluorescent advanced glycosylation end products in collagen. Cardiovasc Res 1993; 27:942–5.

10. Alteon. [see www.alteonpharma.com].

11. Asif M, Egon J, Vason S, et al. An advanced glycation endproduct cross-link breaker can reverse age-related increases in myocardial stiffness. Proc Natl Acad Sci USA 2000; 97:2809–13.

12. Wolffenbuttel BH, Boulanger CM, Crijns FR, et al. Breakers of advanced glycation end products restore large artery properties in experimental diabetes. Proc Natl Acad Sci USA 1998; 95:4630–4.

13. Kass DA, Shapiro EP, Kawaguchi M, et al. Improved arterial compliance by a novel advanced glycation end-product crosslink breaker. Circulation 2001; 104:1464–70.

14. Greene DA, Lattimer SA, Sima AA. Sorbitol, phosphoinositides, and sodium–potassium–ATPase in the pathogenesis of diabetic complications. New Engl J Med 1987; 316:599–606.

15. Tomlinson DR, Dewhurst M, Stevens EJ, et al. Reduced nerve blood flow in diabetic rats: relationship to nitric oxide production and inhibition of aldose reductase. Diabet Med 1998; 15:579–85.

16. Richard S, Tamas C, Sell DR, Monnier VM. Tissue-specific effects of aldose reductase inhibition on fluorescence and cross-linking of extracellular matrix in chronic galactosemia. Relationship to pentosidine cross-links. Diabetes 1991; 40:1049–56.

17. Dunlop M. Aldose reductase and the role of the polyol pathway in diabetic nephropathy. Kidney Int 2000; 58:3–12.

18. Ishii H, Jirousek MR, Koya D, et al. Amelioration of vascular dysfunctions in diabetic rats by an oral PKC beta inhibitor. Science 1996; 272:728–31.

19. Chaturvedi N. Modulation of the renin–angiotensin system and retinopathy. Heart 2000; 84(Suppl 1); 29–31:discussion 50.

20. Leehey DJ, Singh AK, Alavi N, Singh R. Role of angiotensin II in diabetic nephropathy. Kidney Int 2000; 58:93–8.

21. Osicka TM, Yu Y, Lee V, et al. Aminoguanidine and ramipril prevent diabetes-induced increases in protein kinase C activity in glomeruli, retina and mesenteric artery. Clin Sci (Colch) 2001; 100:249–57.

22. Gilbert RE, Kelly DJ, Cox AJ, et al. Angiotensin converting enzyme inhibition reduces retinal overexpression of vascular endothelial growth factor and hyperpermeability in experimental diabetes. Diabetologia 2000; 43:1360–7.

23. Gilbert RE, Cox A, Wu L, et al. Expression of transforming growth factor-beta1 and type IV collagen in the renal tubulointerstitium in experimental diabetes: effects of ACE inhibition. Diabetes 1998; 47:414–22.

24. Reeves WB, Andreoli TE. Transforming growth factor beta contributes to progressive diabetic nephropathy. Proc Natl Acad Sci USA 2000; 97:7667–9.

25. Ziyadeh FN, Hoffman BB, Han DC, et al. Long-term prevention of renal insufficiency, excess matrix gene expression, and glomerular mesangial matrix expansion by treatment with monoclonal anti-transforming growth factor-beta antibody in db/db diabetic mice. Proc Natl Acad Sci USA 2000; 97:8015–20.

26. Aiello LP, Wong JS. Role of vascular endothelial growth factor in diabetic vascular complications. Kidney Int 2000; 58:113–19.

27. Aiello LP. Eye complications of diabetes. In: Khan RC, editor. Atlas of diabetes. London: Scientific Press; 2000:135–49.

28. Michaelson IC. The mode of development of the vascular system of the retina, with some observations on its significance for certain retinal diseases. Trans Opthalmol Soc UK 1948; 68: 137–80.

29. Stratton IM, Kohner EM, Aldington SJ, et al. UKPDS 50: risk factors for incidence and progression of retinopathy in type II diabetes over 6 years from diagnosis. Diabetologia 2001; 44:156–63.

30. Cohen RA, Hennekens CH, Christen WG, et al. Determinants of retinopathy progression in type 1 diabetes mellitus. Am J Med 1999; 107:45–51.

31. The EUCLID Study Group. Randomised placebo-controlled trial of lisinopril in normotensive patients with insulin-dependent diabetes and normoalbuminuria or microalbuminuria. Lancet 1997; 349:1787–92.

32. UK Prospective Diabetes Study Group. Tight blood pressure control and risk of macrovascular and microvascular complications in type 2 diabetes: UKPDS 38. Br Med J 1998; 317:703–13.

33. Early Treatment Diabetic Retinopathy Study Research Group. Early photocoagulation for diabetic retinopathy. ETDRS report number 9. Ophthalmology 1991; 98:766–85.

34. Aiello LP, Pierce EA, Foley ED, et al. Suppression of retinal neovascularization in vivo by inhibition of vascular endothelial growth factor (VEGF) using soluble VEGF-receptor chimeric proteins. Proc Natl Acad Sci USA 1995; 92:10,457–61.

35. Parving HH, Tarnow L, Rossing P. Genetics of diabetic nephropathy. J Am Soc Nephrol 1996; 7: 2509–17.

36. Kunz R, Bork JP, Fritsche L, et al. Association between the angiotensin-converting enzyme – insertion/deletion polymorphism and diabetic nephropathy: a methodologic appraisal and systematic review. J Am Soc Nephrol 1998; 9:1653–63.

37. Bojestig M, Arnqvist HJ, Hermansson G, Karlberg BE, Ludvigsson J. Declining incidence of nephropathy in insulin-dependent diabetes mellitus. New Engl J Med 1994; 330:15–18.

38. Parving HH, Andersen AR, Smidt UM, et al. Effect of antihypertensive treatment on kidney function

in diabetic nephropathy. Br Med J (Clin Res Edn) 1987; 294:1443–7.

39. Ohkubo Y, Kishikawa H, Araki E, et al. Intensive insulin therapy prevents the progression of diabetic microvascular complications in Japanese patients with non-insulin-dependent diabetes mellitus: a randomized prospective 6–year study. Diabetes Res Clin Pract 1995; 28:103–17.

40. Kimmelstiel K, Wilson C. Intercapillary lesions in the glomeruli of the kidney. Am J Path 1936; 12:83–105.

41. The sixth report of the Joint National Committee on prevention, detection, evaluation, and treatment of high blood pressure. Archs Intern Med 1997; 157:2413–46.

42. Kasiske BL, Kalil RS, Ma JZ, et al. Effect of antihypertensive therapy on the kidney in patients with diabetes: a meta-regression analysis. Ann Intern Med 1993; 118:129–38.

43. Bohlen L, de Courten M, Weidmann P. Comparative study of the effect of ACE-inhibitors and other antihypertensive agents on proteinuria in diabetic patients. Am J Hypertens 1994; 7:84S–92S.

44. The ACE inhibitors in Diabetic Nephropathy Trialist Group. Should all patients with type 1 diabetes mellitus and microalbuminuria receive angiotensin-converting enzyme inhibitors? A meta-analysis of individual patient data. Ann Intern Med 2001; 134: 370–9.

45. Marre M, Chatellier G, Leblanc H, et al. Prevention of diabetic nephropathy with enalapril in normotensive diabetics with microalbuminuria. Br Med J 1988; 297: 1092–5.

46. Hallab M, Gallois Y, Chatellier G, et al. Comparison of reduction in microalbuminuria by enalapril and hydrochlorothiazide in normotensive patients with insulin dependent diabetes. Br Med J 1993; 306:175–82.

47. Jerums GAT, Campbell DJ, Cooper ME, et al. Comparison between perindopril and nifedipine in normotensive patients with type 1 diabetes and microalbuminuria. The Melbourne Diabetic Nephropathy Study Group. Am J Kid Dis 2001; 37:890–9.

48. Jerums G, Allen TJ, Gilbert RE, et al. Natural history of early diabetic nephropathy: what are the effects of therapeutic intervention? Melbourne Diabetic Nephropathy Study Group. J Diabetes Complic 1995; 9:308–14.

49. Crepaldi G, Carta Q, Deferrari G, et al. Effects of lisinopril and nifedipine on the progression to overt albuminuria in IDDM patients with incipient nephropathy and normal blood pressure. The Italian Microalbuminuria Study Group in IDDM. Diabetes Care 1998; 21:104–10.

50. Ravid M, Savin H, Jutrin I, et al. Long-term stabilizing effect of angiotensin-converting enzyme inhibition on plasma creatinine and on proteinuria in normotensive type II diabetic patients. Ann Intern Med 1993; 118:577–81.

51. Ravid M, Brosh D, Levi Z, et al. Use of enalapril to attenuate decline in renal function in normotensive, normoalbuminuric patients with type 2 diabetes mellitus. A randomized, controlled trial. Ann Intern Med 1998; 128:982–8.

52. Sano T, Hotta N, Kawamura T, et al. Effects of long-term enalapril treatment on persistent microalbuminuria in normotensive type 2 diabetic patients: results of a 4–year, prospective, randomized study. Diabet Med 1996; 13:120–4.

53. Lewis EJ, Hunsicker LG, Bain RP, Rohde RD. The effect of angiotensin-converting-enzyme

inhibition on diabetic nephropathy. The Collaborative Study Group. New Engl J Med 1993; 329: 1456–62.

54. Hebert LA, Bain RP, Verme D, et al. Remission of nephrotic range proteinuria in type I diabetes. Collaborative Study Group. Kidney Int 1994; 46:1688–93.

55. Brenner BM, Cooper ME, de Zeeuw D, et al. Effects of losartan on renal and cardiovascular outcomes in patients with Type 2 diabetes and nephropathy. N Engl J Med 2001; 345:861–9.

56. Lewis EJ, Hunsicker LG, Clarke WR, et al. Renoprotective effect of the angiotensin – receptor antagonist irbesartan in patients with nephropathy due to Type 2 diabetes. N Engl J Med 2001; 345: 851–60

57. Parving HH, Lehnert H, Brochner-Mortensen J, et al. The effect of irbesartan on the development of diabetic nephropathy in patients with Type 2 diabetes. N Engl J Med 2001; 345:870–8.

58. Park YS, Guijarro C, Kim Y, et al. Lovastatin reduces glomerular macrophage influx and expression of monocyte chemoattractant protein-1 mRNA in nephrotic rats. Am J Kidney Dis 1998; 31:190–4.

59. Hommel E, Andersen P, Gall MA, et al. Plasma lipoproteins and renal function during simvastatin treatment in diabetic nephropathy. Diabetologia 1992; 35:447–51.

60. Tonolo G, Ciccarese M, Brizzi P, et al. Reduction of albumin excretion rate in normotensive microalbuminuric type 2 diabetic patients during long-term simvastatin treatment. Diabetes Care 1997; 20: 1891–5.

61. Thomas PK. Classification, differential diagnosis, and staging of diabetic peripheral neuropathy. Diabetes 1997; 46(Suppl 2): S54–S57.

62. Pirart J. [Degenerative diabetic complications. Is persistent hyperglycemia more dangerous than wide glycemic fluctuations?] Nouv Presse Med 1978; 7:4031–5.

63. Dahl-Jorgensen K. Near-normoglycemia and late diabetic complications. The Oslo Study. Acta Endocr 1987; 284(Suppl):1–38.

64. Solders G, Wilczek H, Gunnarson R, et al. Effects of combined pancreatic and renal transplantation on diabetic neuropathy: a two-year follow-up study. Lancet 1987; 2: 1232–5.

65. Navarro X, Sutherland DE, Kennedy WR. Long-term effects of pancreatic transplantation on diabetic neuropathy. Ann Neurol 1997; 42:727–36.

66. Malik RA. Can diabetic neuropathy be prevented by angiotensin-converting enzyme inhibitors? Ann Med 2000; 32:1–5.

67. Engerman RL, Kern TS, Larson ME. Nerve conduction and aldose reductase inhibition during 5 years of diabetes or galactosaemia in dogs. Diabetologia 1994; 37: 141–4.

68. Nicolucci A, Carinci F, Cavaliere D, et al. A meta-analysis of trials on aldose reductase inhibitors in diabetic peripheral neuropathy. The Italian Study Group. The St Vincent Declaration. Diabet Med 1996; 13:1017–26.

69. Ziegler D, Reljanovic M, Mehnert H, Gries FA. Alpha-lipoic acid in the treatment of diabetic polyneuropathy in Germany: current evidence from clinical trials. Expl Clin Endocr Diabetes 1999; 107: 421–30.

70. Keen H, Payan J, Allawi J, et al. Treatment of diabetic neuropathy with gamma-linolenic acid. The gamma-Linolenic Acid Multicenter Trial Group. Diabetes Care 1993; 16:8–15.

71. Apfel SC, Kessler JA, Adornato

BT, et al. Recombinant human nerve growth factor in the treatment of diabetic polyneuropathy. NGF Study Group. Neurology 1998; 51:695–702.

72. McQuay HJ, Tramer M, Nye BA, et al. A systematic review of antidepressants in neuropathic pain. Pain 1996; 68:217–27.

73. Kiayias JA, Vlachou ED, Lakka-Papadodima E. Venlafaxine HCl in the treatment of painful peripheral diabetic neuropathy. Diabetes Care 2000; 23:699.

74. McQuay H, Carroll D, Jadad AR, et al. Anticonvulsant drugs for management of pain: a systematic review. Br Med J 1995; 311: 1047–52.

75. Backonja M, Beydoun A, Edwards KR, et al. Gabapentin for the symptomatic treatment of painful neuropathy in patients with diabetes mellitus: a randomized controlled trial. J Am Med Ass 1998; 280:1831–6.

76. The Capsaicin Study Group. Treatment of painful diabetic neuropathy with topical capsaicin. A multicenter, double-blind, vehicle-controlled study. Archs Intern Med 1991; 151:2225–9.

77. Biesbroeck R, Bril V, Hollander P, et al. A double-blind comparison of topical capsaicin and oral amitriptyline in painful diabetic neuropathy. Adv Ther 1995; 12: 111–20.

78. Kastrup J, Petersen P, Dejgard A, et al. Intravenous lidocaine infusion – a new treatment of chronic painful diabetic neuropathy? Pain 1987; 28:69–75.

79. Dejgard A, Petersen P, Kastrup J. Mexiletine for treatment of chronic painful diabetic neuropathy. Lancet 1988; 1:9–11.

5
What are the long-term consequences of hypoglycaemia in Type 1 diabetes?

Brian M Frier and Andrew J Sommerfield

Introduction

Insulin replacement is fundamental to the treatment and well-being of people with insulin-deficient diabetes. However, despite refinements in insulin formulations and improved methods of insulin delivery, it is still very difficult to match the administration of exogenous insulin to an individual's energy requirements on a daily basis. Fluctuations in blood glucose are common and occasional hypoglycaemia is almost an inevitable consequence of effective insulin therapy. Not only is hypoglycaemia common, it is the most feared side effect of insulin treatment, and is a major limiting factor to achieving and maintaining good glycaemic control. Although hypoglycaemia can also be associated with sulphonylurea therapy, this occurs much less frequently than insulin-induced hypoglycaemia and is seldom severe.

As a side effect of insulin therapy, severe hypoglycaemia (defined as any episode requiring external assistance for recovery) is not trivial and must not be dismissed by physicians as an unavoidable nuisance. It is extremely unpleasant, associated with acute and chronic morbidity of a serious nature,[1] can impinge on every aspect of everyday life, and may occasionally be fatal. The Diabetes Control and Complications Trial (DCCT)[2] and the Stockholm Diabetes Intervention Study (SDIS)[3] clearly demonstrated that strict glycaemic control in people with Type 1 diabetes is pursued at the price of exposure to a higher frequency of severe hypoglycaemia. Current therapeutic policies that encourage patients to achieve continuous normoglycaemia with intensive insulin regimens, and the expanding use of insulin in the management of Type 2 diabetes, are likely to promote more frequent hypoglycaemic events of varying severity. Recurrent exposure to severe hypoglycaemia may have serious long-term consequences for individual patients and it is axiomatic that its frequency must be kept to a minimum. A wider acceptance by physicians of the potential risks associated with hypoglycaemia should influence modern therapeutic strategies for the clinical management of diabetes.

Physiological responses to hypoglycaemia

The human brain is dependent upon glucose as its main source of energy and rapidly malfunctions if deprived of this substrate. To protect the function and integrity of the central nervous system, and to restore homeostasis as rapidly as possible, a hierarchy of responses are activated when blood glucose falls below 4.0mmol/l. These incorporate diverse biochemical and physiological changes that strive to restore blood glucose concentration to normal, and so reduce the risk of protracted neuroglycopenia. The secretion of counterregulatory hormones, the onset of autonomic symptoms and the development of cognitive dysfunction are triggered when the blood glucose declines to specific blood glucose concentrations, or glycaemic thresholds; these concentrations are reproducible within individuals but can be modified by extraneous factors, such as the prevailing degree of glycaemic control in people with diabetes.

Animal studies suggest that counterregulatory responses are initiated by the stimulation of putative glucose sensors within the central nervous system (principally the hypothalamus), and through a peripheral sensor mechanism in the portal vein.[4] In addition, glucopenia appears to have a direct effect on the pancreatic islets to promote glucagon secretion. Counterregulatory responses are mediated by neural stimulation, provoking the release of several hormones, of which glucagon and adrenaline are the most potent in their capacity to mobilize glucose through hepatic glycogenolysis and the synthesis of glucose (gluconeogenesis) in the liver and kidney.[5,6]

Activation of the autonomic nervous system, via hypothalamic autonomic centres, is a prominent manifestation of the integrated response to hypoglycaemia, stimulating the peripheral sympatho–adrenal system and causing a profuse secretion of adrenaline equivalent to that observed in major medical emergencies, such as acute myocardial infarction. While adrenaline has a prominent counterregulatory role, it also augments physiological changes that occur as a consequence of autonomic arousal. These generate subjective sensations that are interpreted within the brain as symptoms of hypoglycaemia. In addition, catecholamines have haemodynamic and haemostatic effects. Other hormones that are secreted in response to hypoglycaemia, such as vasopressin and angiotensin II, may contribute to regional and local circulatory changes.

Acute hypoglycaemia provokes pronounced haemodynamic changes that include an increase in heart rate, stroke volume, myocardial contractility and cardiac output, and widening of pulse pressure.[7,8] Regional changes in circulation occur during hypoglycaemia to increase the blood flow to organs such as the brain, liver and skeletal muscle, while perfusion of the kidneys and spleen is reduced.[8] Within the brain, blood flow is increased to the frontal lobes and cortex, and is diminished in some pos-

Table 5.1 Effects of hypoglycaemia on peripheral blood.

Increased white blood cell count (neutrophils and lymphocytes)	Increased haematocrit
Increased platelet activation and aggregation	Elevated red blood cell count
Increased von Willebrand factor	Increased haemoglobin concentration
Increased factor VIII activity	Reduced plasma volume
Elevated fibrinogen concentration	Increased red blood cell aggregation
Increased free radicals	

terior areas. This regional redistribution of the cerebral circulation presumably represents the evolution of a protective response to limit the effects of neuroglycopenia on the most vulnerable parts of the central nervous system.[9] Acute hypoglycaemia also has significant, albeit transient, effects on peripheral blood (Table 5.1), which encourage haemostasis and increase blood viscosity.[8,10] These changes during hypoglycaemia influence capillary blood flow and, in some tissues, may predispose to intravascular stasis.

Although the haemodynamic and haematological changes that occur during acute hypoglycaemia are transient, in terms of intensity and magnitude of effect, they are not minor. While they do not appear to compromise vascular perfusion in the normal healthy vasculature, they may have potentially adverse effects in people with diabetes, in whom endothelial dysfunction and vascular abnormalities are common, with premature atherosclerosis compromising tissue perfusion.

Short-term clinical effects and morbidity of hypoglycaemia

Where vascular function and the circulation to major organs (such as the myocardium) or within vital organs (such as the brain) are already abnormal and diminished, the responses to acute hypoglycaemia may exert pathophysiological effects that manifest as symptoms of localized ischaemia, or may present as specific clinical syndromes.

Cardiovascular events (Table 5.2)

The brief, but intense, haemodynamic response that occurs secondary to the profound sympatho–adrenal activation provoked by hypoglycaemia may precipitate an acute vascular event or a dysrhythmia[8,11] in people who have pre-existing coronary heart disease, or may compromise myocardial contractility in people who have the specific heart disease of

Table 5.2 Cardiovascular effects of acute hypoglycaemia.

Physiological changes	Potential pathological sequelae
Increased heart rate Widening of pulse pressure Increased cardiac output Electrophysiological changes (QT lengthening)	Silent myocardial ischaemia Angina; myocardial infarction Arrhythmias Acute congestive cardiac failure (pulmonary oedema)

diabetes. The increase in plasma adrenaline causes a rapid fall in plasma potassium,[12] which could affect the heart by promoting prolongation of ventricular repolarization. Electrocardiographic changes, including prolongation of the QT interval, T wave flattening and inversion, and ST segment depression, have been demonstrated during experimentally induced hypoglycaemia,[13] and transient cardiac arrhythmias have occasionally been demonstrated in non-diabetic and diabetic subjects during hypoglycaemia.[11] These electrophysiological changes may lead to the generation of a serious cardiac arrhythmia, especially in the presence of occult ischaemic heart disease. Angina, myocardial infarction and acute cardiac failure have also been documented, albeit infrequently and anecdotally, as the direct consequences of acute hypoglycaemia.[11,14] The true incidence of these events is unknown but may be underestimated in clinical practice because the precipitating factor of acute hypoglycaemia is either overlooked, may already have been treated, or counterregulation may have raised blood glucose by the time the patient receives medical attention. These outcomes are more likely to occur in older people who have established macro- and microvascular disease.

Physical injury

Physical injury occurring as a result of severe hypoglycaemia is relatively common. In a retrospective survey of people with insulin-treated diabetes,[1] approximately 10% had suffered a physical injury related to hypoglycaemia at some time during their treatment with insulin. These included skeletal injuries, with fractures and joint dislocations, head injuries and burns, in addition to the more frequent minor soft tissue injuries of bruises, cuts and lacerations. Injuries may occur as a result of falls following dizziness, incoordination, drowsiness, loss of consciousness or convulsions,[15] and may be the consequence of road traffic accidents caused by hypoglycaemia.

Cerebral events

In humans, the most important organ to be affected by acute hypoglycaemia is the brain. Progressive neuroglycopenia causes cognitive impairment,[16,17] manifested initially as difficulty concentrating and reduced speed of intellectual functioning, but proceeding to drowsiness, confusion and, ultimately, loss of consciousness. Mood changes are common and include tense-tiredness, anger, depression, anxiety and pessimism.[17] Denial of hypoglycaemia is common, behavioural change may sometimes occur with irrational and aggressive responses, and occasionally a state of automatism may develop. Recovery is usually rapid after the blood glucose concentration returns to normal. Most aspects of intellectual function recover within 45–90 minutes,[18,19] and even after an episode of severe hypoglycaemic coma, recovery is complete within 24 hours.[20] However, disturbance of mood and memory, and a feeling of general malaise, may persist for longer,[20] and amnesia of severe hypoglycaemia is common.

Electrophysiological manifestations of cerebral dysfunction accompany the cognitive and mood changes. Characteristic electroencephalographic (EEG) changes occur during acute hypoglycaemia in the waking state. A decrease in alpha waves is accompanied by an increase in delta and theta waves, which are more pronounced over anterior parts of the brain.[21,22] These changes are more prominent in people with Type 1 diabetes – EEG evidence of epileptiform activity during hypoglycaemia has been recorded more commonly in these subjects than in non-diabetic persons.[23] Acute neuroglycopenia is a recognized cause of focal or generalized convulsions, and in an individual treated with insulin it is important to exclude acute hypoglycaemia as a cause of a seizure. Transient hemiplegia is another manifestation of acute hypoglycaemia,[24] although it is unclear whether the mechanism is the direct effect of neuroglycopenia or whether altered regional blood flow causes localized ischaemia within the brain. In older persons, acute changes in regional cerebrovascular perfusion may precipitate an acute vascular event such as a transient ischaemic attack or even a stroke.

Coma

Coma is relatively uncommon and constitutes about one third of all episodes of severe hypoglycaemia. Fortunately, prolonged neuroglycopenia associated with hypoglycaemic coma is rare but, when it is associated with the development of cerebral oedema, the mortality is high. Most fatal cases, or those with severe brain damage, follow a deliberate overdose of insulin in an individual with suicidal intent[25] or are associated with the ingestion of an excessive quantity of alcohol.[26] Rarely, deliberate criminal intent is uncovered that then requires careful forensic investigation. The few individuals who survive such protracted, profound neuroglycopenia usually have extensive and permanent neurological damage, associated with severe cognitive impairment and memory loss, and may remain in a chronic vegetative state.[27] In cases with such a disastrous outcome, neuroimaging usually demonstrates cortical and hippocampal atrophy with secondary ventricular enlargement.

Mechanisms of hypoglycaemia-induced brain injury may involve the following:

1   neurochemical changes – hypoglycaemia can cause neuronal death by the release of neuro-excitatory amino acids, such as glutamate and aspartate, which are neurotoxic;[28,29]
2   neuronal susceptibility to neuroglycopenia – in humans, the duration of severe hypoglycaemia is probably more important than the depth in causing damage to the brain. Neuropathological observations have confirmed the rostrocaudal direction of vulnerability of the brain to neuroglycopenia. The cerebral cortex and hippocampus are most sensitive, while the hindbrain and spinal cord are relatively resistant to neuroglycopenia.[30,31] This is consistent with clinical experience, which suggests that the higher centres in the brain are affected by lesser degrees of neuroglycopenia;
3   localised cerebral ischaemia – as noted earlier, acute changes in cerebral blood flow during hypoglycaemia have a regional redistribution with a preferential increase in blood flow to the frontal lobes[9]; these changes may induce localized areas of ischaemia in the brain, especially in the presence of cerebrovascular disease.

Fortunately, despite the relative frequency of severe hypoglycaemia, the effects on cerebral function are usually transient and reversible, with only a few anecdotal instances where an isolated episode of profound and prolonged hypoglycaemia has been associated with permanent neurological and/or cognitive dysfunction. In a few individuals with insulin-treated diabetes, a specific and limited neurological deficit has been associated with preceding hypoglycaemia, accompanied by neuroradiological evidence of a localized lesion (Figure 5.1).[24,32,33]

Mortality associated with severe hypoglycaemia

In many surveys, severe hypoglycaemia has been implicated in 2-4% of deaths in the insulin-treated diabetic population.[34,35] The number is difficult to estimate with accuracy because of the problems associated with identifying and confirming hypoglycaemia-induced death,[34] and hypoglycaemia may be overlooked as the precipitating factor of a fatal acute vascular event. The risk of sudden death in people with insulin-dependent diabetes is higher than that of a non-diabetic population of equivalent age; in younger people this is principally attributable to metabolic causes, including severe hypoglycaemia.[35]

Hypoglycaemia has been implicated in the 'dead in bed' syndrome,[36–39] in which young people with insulin-treated diabetes, who have

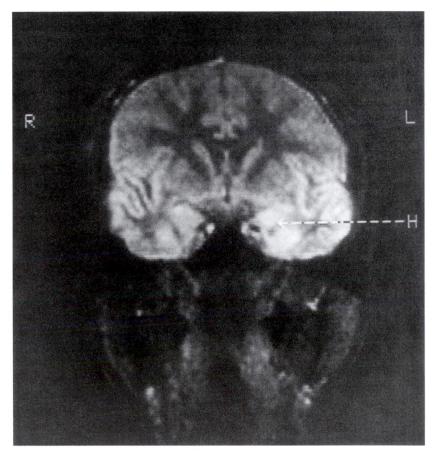

Figure 5.1

MRI scan (T1-weighted) showing high signal areas in the left hippocampus in a man with Type 1 diabetes following an episode of hypoglycaemic coma. He subsequently had evidence of memory loss. From Chalmers *et al.*,[32] with the permission of the American Diabetes Association.

been in good health and have been sleeping alone, are found dead in an undisturbed bed. 'Dead in bed' syndrome accounts for 6% of deaths amongst individuals with Type 1 diabetes under 40 years of age, occurring at a rate of two to six events per 100,000 patient years.[39] Hypoglycaemia-induced cardiac arrhythmia, acute respiratory arrest with impaired baroreflex sensitivity[40] and undetected autonomic dysfunction,[41] have all been suggested as possible causative mechanisms. The sudden development of a fatal cardiac arrhythmia is the more likely explanation, as death from neuroglycopenic cerebral damage is relatively slow and is accompanied by characteristic neuropathological changes. In fatal cases of hypoglycaemia, the histopathology of the brain is very variable,[31] depending upon the clinical course and whether the fatal outcome was complicated by the development of convulsions, pulmonary aspiration or respiratory infection (causing hypoxia) during the terminal illness.

Long-term effects of recurrent hypoglycaemia

It is evident that isolated episodes of severe hypoglycaemia can have long-term sequelae in terms of permanent neurological deficit, cognitive impairment, irreversible EEG abnormalities or the outcome of a vascular event or injury. However, recurrent exposure to hypoglycaemia of variable severity may have more subtle and insidious deleterious effects on intellectual function, and may be responsible for the development of acquired hypoglycaemia syndromes such as impaired awareness of hypoglycaemia, counterregulatory deficiencies or hypoglycaemia-induced autonomic failure.

Impaired cognitive function

In recent years, evidence has accumulated to suggest that diabetes per se may be associated with the gradual emergence of modest cognitive impairment.[42–45] This presumably develops as a result of prolonged exposure to hyperglycaemia and other metabolic abnormalities, and is compounded by the effects of hypertension and vascular disease on the brain. Potential causes of cognitive impairment in diabetes are listed in Table 5.3. Among these, repeated exposure to severe hypoglycaemia has been postulated to cause progressive cognitive dysfunction in some people with Type 1 diabetes. This premise is controversial and is therefore reviewed in some detail.

Occasional non-diabetic patients who have been subjected to chronic neuroglycopenia as a result of an insulinoma have been reported to develop significant and permanent deterioration in intellectual function.[47] Anecdotal case reports in people with insulin-treated diabetes have

Table 5.3 Possible causes of cognitive impairment in diabetes.

Chronic hyperglycaemia
Recurrent severe hypoglycaemia
Cerebrovascular disease; ischaemia, infarction
Recurrent diabetic ketoacidosis
Depression; psychiatric disorders
Hypertension
Psychosocial impact of chronic disease
Alcohol, drug abuse

suggested that recurrent exposure to severe hypoglycaemia may have lasting consequences, resulting in a chronic deterioration of cognitive function with reduced intellectual ability, impaired social skills and behaviour, inability to maintain employment and increasing dependence on a spouse or carer.[48] The age of onset of diabetes is an important determinant of the potential effects that recurrent hypoglycaemia may have on cognitive function and intellectual ability, with children being the most susceptible.

Effects of recurrent hypoglycaemia in childhood

The developing and immature brain of the young child is particularly vulnerable to the effects of neuroglycopenia. The deleterious influence of hypoglycaemia on intellect and cerebral function has been shown to be greatest in children who have developed diabetes before 5 years of age and who have been exposed to multiple episodes of severe hypoglycaemia in early childhood, especially when these have provoked convulsions.[49–52] Cognitive dysfunction may become manifest later in childhood or adolescence with demonstrable learning difficulties, and occasionally with abnormal behaviour.[52]

Several retrospective, cross-sectional[49,50] and prospective studies[53,54] have shown an association between the early onset of Type 1 diabetes in childhood and lower than expected powers of attention and psychomotor efficiency in adolescence, when compared to non-diabetic peer groups.[55] A direct correlation has been demonstrated between the frequency of hypoglycaemia-induced convulsions at this age and evidence of cognitive dysfunction later in life.[52,54–56] Children with onset of diabetes after 5 years of age also perform less well than their non-diabetic peer group on many tests of cognitive function, especially on assessment of verbal IQ. However, this is considered to be a consequence of the psychosocial and educational effects of diabetes, with factors such as interrupted school attendance through ill health or intermittent metabolic disturbances playing a significant role, rather than a direct pathophysiological effect of repetitive hypoglycaemia on the brain.[52]

Effects of recurrent hypoglycaemia in adulthood

The relationship between cognitive dysfunction and the frequency of exposure to severe hypoglycaemia has been examined in adults with insulin-treated diabetes, but with less definitive results than those observed in children. Two major prospective studies, the DCCT[57] and the SDIS,[58] have not shown an association between the frequency of severe hypoglycaemia and measures of cognitive function.[59] Both of these studies were designed to evaluate the effect of strict glycaemic control on limiting the complications of diabetes. The participants were subdivided into intensively treated and conventionally treated subgroups, achieving strict or moderate glycaemic control, respectively; the incidence and progression of diabetic complications and the frequency of adverse effects of treatment were monitored prospectively. Both studies have shown unequivocally that strict glycaemic control limits the development and progression of diabetic microangiopathy, but is accompanied by a higher rate of severe hypoglycaemia.

In the DCCT, a comprehensive battery of tests of cognitive function was applied, whereas the cognitive tests used in the SDIS were much more limited, and a clear separation of the groups was not achieved in terms of exposure to severe hypoglycaemia.[58] However, in both studies, the higher frequency of severe hypoglycaemia in the patients with strict glycaemic control was not associated with any evidence of intellectual decline.

While these results are reassuring and suggest that mental ability is not being affected adversely by repeated exposure to severe hypoglycaemia, they need to be interpreted with caution. Both the DCCT and SDIS had stringent recruitment criteria. The participants, and the extent of medical support available to them, were not representative of the insulin-treated diabetic population in general. They were relatively young and had diabetes of short duration. They were above average intelligence, many were highly motivated and well educated in self-care of their diabetes. People who had a history of multiple episodes of severe hypoglycaemia were excluded. This criterion is likely to have excluded anyone with impaired hypoglycaemia awareness, so that few, if any, patients who were recruited to participate in these studies were at high risk of developing severe hypoglycaemia. It would be imprudent, therefore, to extrapolate the conclusions from these studies to the archetypal population with Type 1 diabetes, which is much more heterogeneous, and includes people who have impaired awareness of hypoglycaemia and other risk factors for severe hypoglycaemia. The rate of severe hypoglycaemia in unselected populations is double that observed in the DCCT group who had strict glycaemic control.[1,60] Furthermore, cognitive decline may be a late manifestation of the cumulative effects of severe hypoglycaemia, emerging after 20 years or more of treatment with insulin, and the causes may be multifactorial. The timescale of the follow-up (< 10 years) of these two major prospective studies may not have been long enough to reveal the development of an intellectual deficit.

By contrast, studies in adult patients with Type 1 diabetes that have relied on a retrospective estimate of the frequency of exposure to recurrent severe hypoglycaemia have demonstrated a significant correlation with evidence of impaired intellectual function. In an early study, measures of global intelligence in 100 adults with insulin-treated diabetes were compared with demographically matched, non-diabetic controls.[61] Intellectual function was impaired in the diabetic group compared to the control group and the cognitive decrement appeared to be related to the estimated number and severity of previous episodes of hypoglycaemia.[61] An association between the estimated number of previous severe hypoglycaemic events and the neuropsychological test performance of adults with Type 1 diabetes has been observed in other studies.[62,63] In a Swedish study of a small group of 17 adults with Type 1 diabetes, all of whom had a history of recurrent severe hypoglycaemia, deficits were demonstrated in tests of problem solving, motor ability, visuospatial skills and in tasks that assess frontal lobe functions.[63] However, the study design did not preclude the possibility that the patients who had a history of recurrent hypoglycaemia may have been those who had a lower pre-morbid IQ and, being less adept in their self-management of diabetes, had therefore experienced a higher frequency of severe hypoglycaemia.

This possibility was avoided in a study in Edinburgh,[64] in which the degree of intellectual impairment was estimated as the difference between measures of premorbid and current IQ. A significant correlation was demonstrated between the degree of cognitive impairment and the frequency of severe hypoglycaemia in a group of 100 adults who had developed Type 1 diabetes in adulthood (i.e. after full maturation of the brain and attainment of intellectual ability). Partial correlation analysis showed that the observed correlations were not related to age, duration of diabetes or blood glucose measured at the time of cognitive testing. The group could be divided approximately into quartiles on the basis of their previous experience of severe hypoglycaemia. These subgroups were matched for age, duration of diabetes, education, social class and premorbid IQ. Comparison of the quartile who had a history of five or more episodes of severe hypoglycaemia with the quartile with no previous severe hypoglycaemia, revealed significant differences in IQ deficit (Figure 5.2), performance IQ and reaction time.[64] Individual differences in

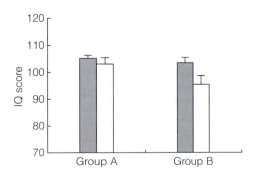

Figure 5.2

Comparison of premorbid (solid bars) and present (open bars) IQ levels between a group of individuals with Type 1 diabetes with no history of previous severe hypoglycaemia (group A) and a group of individuals with Type 1 diabetes with a history of at least five previous episodes of severe hypoglycemia (group B). Premorbid versus present IQ comparison for group A is not significant, for group B it is significant at p < 0.001. Reproduced from Langan *et al.*,[64] with the permission of Diabetologia.

the experience of severe hypoglycaemia were not related to differences in premorbid intelligence.

While this study indicated a relationship between the frequency of severe hypoglycaemia and cognitive impairment,[64] it could not exclude the possibility that diabetes per se was influencing cognitive function. The subjects with Type 1 diabetes were therefore compared with a group of non-diabetic controls, matched for premorbid IQ, age and educational experience. This demonstrated that the performance and verbal IQs of the diabetic participants were lower than the non-diabetic controls.[65] Within the group of subjects with diabetes, the effect of previous severe hypoglycaemia was associated specifically with a deficit in performance IQ, and decision making and response initiation skills were affected adversely in preference to processes that involved the encoding and storage of information.[66] The lower verbal IQ in the subjects with Type 1 diabetes may therefore be the consequence of other factors, such as the social and educational impact of having this disorder. A different study, which used an identical protocol and selection criteria for a group of 70 subjects with Type 1 diabetes, was subsequently performed in Nottingham and reported very similar findings.[67]

These studies have shown the existence of a positive correlation between the frequency of severe hypoglycaemia and a modest degree of intellectual impairment. Although the mean decrement in intellectual ability resulting from recurrent severe hypoglycaemia in the Edinburgh study[64–66] was small (approximately 6 IQ points), this deficit is significant (equivalent to half a standard deviation) and potentially important. It would be sufficient to influence competence in tasks that require intellectual dexterity and could adversely affect individuals who have intellectually demanding occupations, in terms of job performance and capability. While this mean decrement represented the average effect of recurrent severe hypoglycaemia on performance IQ in the group, some individuals were affected to a greater degree. It is also pertinent to emphasize that the participants had developed Type 1 diabetes in adulthood, after full intellectual ability had been achieved, and that very strict inclusion criteria were applied to avoid confounding variables that could have affected cognitive function adversely, such as hypertension, previous head injury, psychiatric illness and alcohol abuse. In most people with Type 1 diabetes, the modest cognitive deficits indicated by the retrospective studies are unlikely to be obvious in the performance of everyday tasks, as the decline in intellectual function is small and appears to be slowly progressive. In older people intellectual decline may be attributed to the ageing process and disregarded.

While these retrospective studies suggest that recurrent exposure to severe hypoglycaemia may cause a modest decline in cognitive function, a major criticism is that they are limited by the accuracy of recall of previous hypoglycaemic events. However, in some studies,[64,65,67] the accuracy of individual reporting was enhanced by interviewing relatives and by scrutiny of medical records. In addition, the cohort with Type 1 diabetes in the original Edinburgh study[64] was reassessed within a period of 18 months, and their estimated frequency of severe hypoglycaemia showed good reliability with the rate that had been reported previously,[66] so helping to validate the method used to estimate the frequency of previous severe hypoglycaemia.

A further piece of supportive evidence comes from clinical and experimental observations of people with Type 1 diabetes who have chronic impairment of awareness of hypoglycaemia (see later) who have a high frequency of severe hypoglycaemia. In these individuals cognitive dysfunction is more profound during acute hypoglycaemia,[68,69] and persists for longer following restoration of normoglycaemia than in unaffected people with Type 1 diabetes who have normal awareness of hypoglycaemia. In a population study, a modest decline in intellectual function was noted to be associated with impaired awareness of hypoglycaemia.[70] In addition, a study of the speed of recovery of cognitive function following a single episode of severe hypoglycaemic coma in a group of people with Type 1 diabetes suggested that cognitive decrements and altered mood states in those with a history of recurrent severe hypoglycaemia were persistent, and were probably a consequence of previous repeated exposure to severe neuroglycopenia.[20] This suggests that the frequent exposure to severe hypoglycaemia suffered by people with Type 1 diabetes who have impaired awareness of hypoglycaemia may have a long-term detrimental effect on intellectual function.

In conclusion, it is possible that repeated episodes of severe hypoglycaemia may have a deleterious effect on cognitive function that is cumulative over time and is akin to the chronic intellectual impairment associated with repeated exposure to other acute neurotoxic insults, such as alcohol abuse, hypoxia (sleep apnoea) and repetitive head injury (boxing). Individuals may vary in their susceptibility to hypoglycaemic injury and a wide spectrum of abnormality is likely, with only a few individuals developing severe intellectual impairment.[48] However, although the results of studies are suggestive that recurrent hypoglycaemia in adults may have a deleterious long-term effect on cognitive function, the evidence is still equivocal and remains unproven.

Structural changes in the brain in diabetes: the role of hypoglycaemia
If cognitive impairment is a permanent consequence of recurrent severe hypoglycaemia, could this cause structural changes in the brain in people with diabetes? Most neuroimaging studies of the brain have been performed in people with Type 2 diabetes and have shown that structural degenerative changes are more common than in non-diabetic controls of a similar age.[71] The clinical significance of these neuroimaging abnormalities is not yet known, but is suggestive of a premature ageing of the

brain. Cortical atrophy (Figure 5.3a) is present in 36-53% of subjects with Type 2 diabetes compared to 12% of matched non-diabetic controls, occurs earlier in life and is more extensive in people with diabetes .[71] Leukoaraiosis (Figure 5.3b), a patchy area of either focal or diffuse

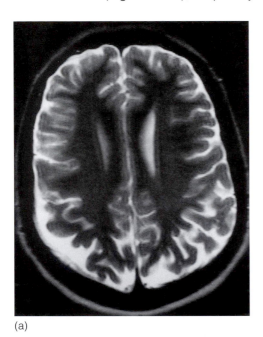

(a)

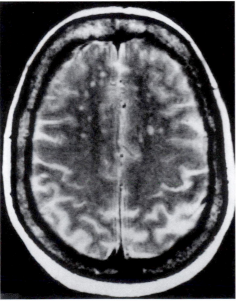

(b)

Figure 5.3

MRI scans demonstrating neurodegenerative changes observed in the brains of patients with Type 1 diabetes. (a) Cortical atrophy; (b) leukoaraiosis. From Hypoglycaemia in clinical diabetes (Frier BM, Fisher BM, editors. Chichester: John Wiley and Sons; 1999), with the permission of the publishers.

demyelination and gliosis, is a non-specific, age-related finding and is associated with several pathological conditions, including hypertension, vascular disease, demyelination and dementia.[72] It has been identified in 69% of subjects with diabetes compared to 12% of non-diabetic controls of similar age.[73] A significantly higher incidence of degenerative changes in the brain has also been reported in subjects with Type 1 diabetes compared to age-matched non-diabetic controls,[74,75] but the cause is unknown.

A few studies have tried to identify whether structural changes in the brains of diabetic subjects are associated with deficits in intellectual performance[76–78] but to date the results have been inconclusive. Magnetic resonance imaging (MRI) scans of the brain were performed in a subgroup of subjects who had participated in the major Edinburgh study described earlier,[64–66] and an association was observed between the presence of cortical atrophy and a history of recurrent severe hypoglycaemia.[75] However, the number of people in this study was too small to demonstrate any significant correlation with impaired cognitive function. Furthermore, it is possible that Type 1 diabetes per se could be an important pathogenetic factor. This premise has been supported by the preliminary results of another large study in the authors' centre of young patients who had developed Type 1 diabetes in childhood or adolescence and in whom any abnormalities, demonstrated by neuroimaging (using MRI), were related to an assessment of their cognitive function.[79] No correlation has been observed between structural changes in the brain and any abnormality of cognitive function, but MRI changes were more common in a subgroup of patients who had diabetic retinopathy. This would suggest that exposure to chronic hyperglycaemia may be of greater importance than hypoglycaemia in causing cerebral changes in young people with Type 1 diabetes. This interpretation is consistent with an earlier American study of young adults with Type 1 diabetes,[80] in whom evidence of impaired cognitive function was associated with peripheral neuropathy (a surrogate marker of chronic hyperglycaemia) and not with previous severe hypoglycaemia per se. However, when the effects of peripheral neuropathy and severe hypoglycaemia were combined, a significant correlation with cognitive dysfunction was observed, suggesting that exposure to severe hypoglycaemia compounds the adverse effect of poor glycaemic control on cerebral function.

It is likely that when cognitive dysfunction does develop in people with insulin-dependent diabetes then this has a multifactorial pathogenesis. Several metabolic factors, including chronic hyperglycaemia (possibly with intermittent exposure to diabetic ketoacidosis) and recurrent hypoglycaemia, may interact to affect neurological function. In addition, evidence is accumulating for the existence of a central neuropathy (or encephalopathy) in people with Type 1 diabetes of long duration,[42–46] which is presumed to have a multifactorial pathogenesis and to which severe hypoglycaemia may contribute.

Acquired hypoglycaemia syndromes

Hypoglycaemia is associated with the development of specific acquired clinical syndromes in Type 1 diabetes and recent research has suggested that these may be the consequences of recurrent exposure to hypoglycaemia per se. They may therefore be regarded as long-term complications of hypoglycaemia.

Impaired awareness of hypoglycaemia

Perception of the onset of warning symptoms of hypoglycaemia is either diminished or absent in approximately 25% of people with insulin-treated diabetes.[81–82] They become unable to detect the early onset of hypoglycaemia, are at an increased risk of recurrent exposure to severe neuroglycopenia and experience a sixfold higher frequency of severe hypoglycaemia.[83] The diminished symptomatic warning of hypoglycaemia should be called 'impaired awareness of hypoglycaemia', as complete loss of awareness is uncommon and most individuals retain a few neuroglycopenic symptoms. Various mechanisms have been proposed to underlie the aetiology of impaired awareness of hypoglycaemia and it is possible that several coexisting factors are important in inducing this condition (Table 5.4). The role of recurrent hypoglycaemia in the development of impaired awareness of hypoglycaemia appears to be of particular importance. Although impaired awareness of hypoglycaemia can be related to the quality of glycaemic control in the short term, it may also be a long-term consequence of recurrent exposure to hypoglycaemia. People with Type 1 diabetes of long duration and who have developed impaired awareness of hypoglycaemia, unrelated to the quality of glycaemic control, have also been shown to have an altered glycaemic threshold for autonomic symptoms, which is set at a lower blood glucose concentration.[68,84] Neuroglycopenia develops before the auto-

Table 5.4 Possible mechanisms of impaired awareness of hypoglycaemia.

Cerebral adaptation
    Strict glycaemic control (HbA$_{1c}$ within non-diabetic range)
    Antecedent hypoglycaemia
    Chronic hypoglycaemia (cf. insulinoma)

CNS glucoregulatory failure
    Counterregulatory deficiency
    Hypoglycaemia-associated central autonomic failure
    Central encephalopathy

Peripheral nervous system dysfunction
    Peripheral autonomic neuropathy
    Reduced peripheral adrenoceptor sensitivity

nomic symptoms, interfering with subjective perceptions of warning symptoms and the ability to self-treat the low blood glucose.

Counterregulatory hormonal deficiencies

The magnitude of counterregulatory hormonal responses to hypoglycaemia declines with increasing duration of diabetes. Hypoglycaemia-induced secretion of glucagon becomes deficient in most people within 5 years of onset of Type 1 diabetes,[85,86] and may be followed within a few years by attenuation of the adrenaline response to hypoglycaemia.[86,87] Diminished hypothalamic–pituitary hormonal secretion in response to hypoglycaemia has also been demonstrated,[88] although the magnitude of the response may be related to the quality of glycaemic control.[89] People with Type 1 diabetes who have counterregulatory deficiencies are at greater risk of experiencing severe hypoglycaemia, particularly if they are subjected to intensive insulin therapy.[90]

In some people with longstanding Type 1 diabetes, peripheral autonomic neuropathy may contribute to a subnormal adrenaline response. However, in most individuals with counterregulatory hormonal deficiencies the blood glucose threshold at which the adrenaline secretory response to hypoglycaemia is triggered has altered such that a lower blood glucose is required to initiate secretion of adrenaline.[91,92] This shift in glycaemic threshold may be a consequence of cerebral adaptation to exposure to recurrent hypoglycaemia.

Cerebral adaptation: altered glycaemic thresholds

The glycaemic thresholds for the development of symptoms of hypoglycaemia and for counterregulatory hormonal secretion are not fixed at a specific blood glucose concentration. In individuals with diabetes, glycaemic thresholds are dynamic and can be influenced by various factors. Cerebral adaptation can occur following short- and longer-term exposure to low blood glucose concentrations, causing elevation of the glycaemic thresholds for secretion of counterregulatory hormones and the onset of symptoms of hypoglycaemia (i.e. a more profound hypoglycaemic stimulus is required). Strict glycaemic control alters the blood glucose thresholds at which the symptomatic and counterregulatory hormonal responses to hypoglycaemia are initiated, so that a lower blood glucose is required to trigger these responses.[93–95] The putative mechanism appears to be an ability of the brain to adapt to function normally in the face of chronic exposure to low blood glucose concentrations. This has been demonstrated in non-diabetic subjects under experimental conditions[96] and in people with Type 1 diabetes who have strict glycaemic control.[97] Attenuation of the neuroendocrine and symptomatic responses occurs in Type 1 diabetes when the glycated haemoglobin HbA_{1C} is within, or near to, the non-diabetic range.[98] Such patients can maintain normal glucose uptake by the brain during hypoglycaemia,[97] so

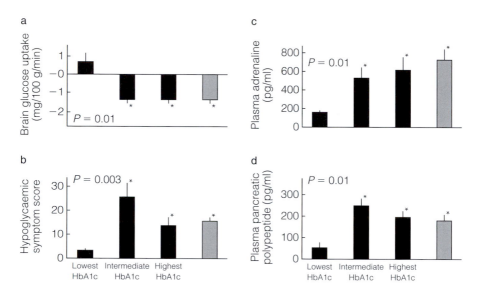

Figure 5.4

Comparison of the changes from baseline in: (a) glucose uptake in the brain;
(b) hypoglycaemia symptom scores; and plasma concentrations of adrenaline (c) and
pancreatic polypeptide (d) during hypoglycaemia in individuals with Type 1 diabetes with
differing degrees of glycaemic control (dark bars) and non-diabetic individuals (light bar).
From Boyle et al.,[97] with the permission of the New England Journal of Medicine.

preserving cerebral metabolism, reducing the neuroendocrine responses
to hypoglycaemia and diminishing symptomatic awareness (Figure 5.4).
Although this protects the brain from the effects of neuroglycopenia, this
is thought to be a maladaptive change, as it suppresses the normal
symptomatic warning, narrows the margin for corrective action to be
taken and so risks the development of more severe neuroglycopenia. In
people with well-controlled Type 2 diabetes (on diet or oral hypoglycaemic agents) the counterregulatory and symptomatic responses
occurred at higher blood glucose concentrations than in non-diabetic
controls.[99] This observation would suggest that the nature of the cerebral
adaptation to strict glycaemic control may be partly related to the form of
treatment employed and that the use of insulin therapy may be responsible for the maladaptive changes in Type 1 diabetes.

The glycaemic threshold for cognitive dysfunction is probably also susceptible to cerebral adaptation, but this remains controversial. Some
studies of people with Type 1 diabetes have shown that, despite strict
glycaemic control or exposure to antecedent hypoglycaemia, cognitive
function remains preserved during experimental hypoglycaemia, with a
shift in the glycaemic threshold for the onset of cognitive dysfunc-

tion.[100–104] However, in other studies, cerebral adaptation to protect cognitive function did not appear to occur and it became impaired at the same blood glucose threshold, irrespective of preceding glycaemic experience.[95,105–108] Thus, in people with Type 1 diabetes who have strict glycaemic control, it remains debatable as to whether the glycaemic threshold for the development of cognitive impairment shifts in parallel with those for the onset of neuroendocrine and symptomatic responses to hypoglycaemia to lower blood glucose concentrations. It has been suggested that a differential change may occur in the blood glucose threshold so that the degree of neuroglycopenia required to compromise intellectual function is less than that needed to generate symptoms and promote effective counterregulation.[109,110] Such an outcome would allow cognitive dysfunction to occur at a higher plasma glucose concentration than that required to trigger the warning symptoms, thereby increasing the risk of severe neuroglycopenia and limiting the scope for intensive insulin therapy.

A single protracted episode of hypoglycaemia, lasting for more than 1 hour, is associated with a diminished magnitude of the symptomatic and neuroendocrine responses to a further episode of hypoglycaemia occurring within the ensuing 48 hours (Figure 5.5).[92,101,111,112] A preceding (antecedent) episode of hypoglycaemia can also promote cerebral adaptation by altering the glycaemic thresholds for symptomatic and neuroendocrine responses to hypoglycaemia. Recurrent exposure to hypoglycaemia may therefore, through the pathogenetic role of antecedent hypoglycaemia, induce the acquired hypoglycaemia syndromes, with modification of the glycaemic thresholds for symptomatic and neuroendocrine responses occurring as a result of cerebral adaptation.

Cerebral adaptation: altered regional blood flow

A permanent redistribution of regional cerebral blood flow occurs in people with Type 1 diabetes who have a history of recurrent severe hypoglycaemia, with a relative but persistent increase in blood flow to the frontal

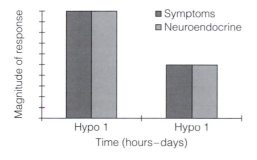

Figure 5.5

Schematic diagram to represent the effect of antecedent hypoglycaemia on symptomatic and neuroendocrine responses to subsequent episodes of hypoglycaemia. From Hypoglycaemia in clinical diabetes (Frier BM, Fisher BM, editors. Chichester: John Wiley and Sons; 1999), with the permission of the publishers.

lobes,[113] which mirrors the normal physiological response to hypogly-caemia.[9] This may represent a chronic adaptive response to protect the most vulnerable parts of the brain from the effects of further severe hypo-glycaemia. However, it has been observed that the changes in regional cerebral blood flow in response to controlled hypoglycaemia occur inde-pendently of the state of awareness of hypoglycaemia in people with Type 1 diabetes,[114] so this is presumably an adaptive response to hypo-glycaemia per se.

Hypoglycaemia-associated autonomic failure

Cryer[115] has suggested that the acquired hypoglycaemia syndromes rep-resent a form of 'hypoglycaemia-associated autonomic failure' (Figure 5.6), implicating recurrent severe hypoglycaemia as the central problem that causes the development of these clinical syndromes. He argues that recurrent exposure to severe hypoglycaemia promotes cerebral adapta-tion, with the resultant alteration of glycaemic thresholds, and the emer-gence of counterregulatory hormonal deficiencies and sympatho–adrenal

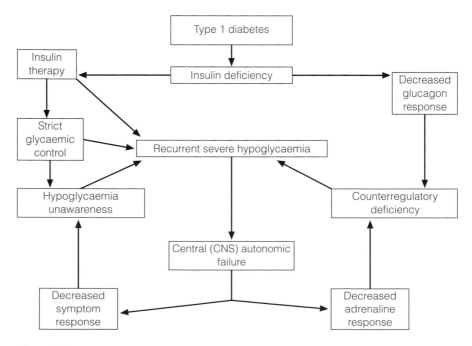

Figure 5.6

Schematic diagram to demonstrate the model of hypoglycaemia-associated autonomic failure, derived from Cryer[115] from Hypoglycaemia in clinical diabetes (Frier BM, Fisher BM, editors. Chichester: John Wiley and Sons; 1999), with the permission of the publishers.

insufficiency, culminating in a chronically impaired awareness of hypo-glycaemia. Repetitive episodes of hypoglycaemia may lead to 'downreg-ulation' of the central mechanisms that normally would respond to a low blood glucose to activate glucoregulatory responses and produce the warning symptoms of hypoglycaemia. As a result, a vicious circle may be established, so that hypoglycaemia promotes further episodes of severe hypoglycaemia, so perpetuating the problem. Scrupulous avoidance of hypoglycaemia for several weeks appears to reverse these effects, at least in part,[116–118] and this has been recommended as a therapeutic strategy to reverse impaired hypoglycaemia awareness. Needless to say, this is very difficult to achieve in clinical practice, but may be assisted by the development of new treatments and technology such as a wider range of insulin analogues, effective insulin pumps and continuous blood glucose monitoring.

Potential effect on microvascular disease

Microvascular disease specific to diabetes takes several years to develop and the principal pathogenetic factor is exposure to chronic hyperglycaemia. It is unlikely that the short-term metabolic abnormalities provoked by acute hypoglycaemia would initiate the development of dia-betic microangiopathy. However, it has been postulated that established microvascular disease is vulnerable to the transient pathophysiological responses induced by acute hypoglycaemia.[119] Thus, a further possible long-term, but hypothetical, effect of recurrent episodes of acute hypo-glycaemia is the possible effect of the haemodynamic and haemostatic changes on established microvascular disease.[8] As stated earlier, the profuse secretion of vasoactive hormones, such as adrenaline, vaso-pressin and angiotensin II, in response to hypoglycaemia can affect the microcirculation. In people with diabetes this may damage capillaries that are already abnormal and have functional effects on vascular flow. The sudden changes in arterial pressure and capillary blood flow may expose the microvasculature to fluctuating stress of varying magnitude. This, in combination with increased plasma viscosity and coagulability, may affect the capillary circulation, reducing capillary blood flow, and encouraging stasis, thrombosis and capillary closure, so producing local-ized ischaemia and hypoxia in vulnerable tissues such as the retina and renal glomeruli. This may lead to capillary closure in tissues already affected by diabetic microvascular disease.

This concept is partly supported by the outcome of studies from the 1980s, including the Kroc, Steno and Oslo studies, which evaluated the effects of rapid improvement in glycaemic control in people with long-standing Type 1 diabetes who had established background diabetic retinopathy.[120] The attainment of strict glycaemic control using intensive insulin therapy did promote an increased frequency of hypoglycaemia and was associated with a rapid worsening of retinopathy within the first 3 months of intensive insulin treatment. While the principal cause for the development of retinal ischaemia during strict glycaemic control was presumed to be the rapid reduction in the retinal hyperperfusion, which is associated with chronic hyperglycaemia, it is tempting to speculate that recurrent acute hypoglycaemia could have had a contributory role.

Anecdotal reports have associated nocturnal hypoglycaemia with acute vitreous haemorrhage in patients who had untreated proliferative diabetic retinopathy.[121,122] The cause may be related to the sudden fall in intra-ocular pressure that occurs in response to acute hypoglycaemia,[123] with the effects of sudden mechanical stress and changes in perfusion pressure, causing rupture of delicate new vessels in the retina and vitreous humour. Hypoglycaemia also causes an acute reduction in renal plasma flow and glomerular filtration,[124] and theoretically may influence progression of glomerular and arteriolar sclerosis in patients with diabetic nephropathy, although at present there is no evidence to support this premise.

Thus, it is hypothetically possible that the sudden haemodynamic changes, and the effects on haemoconcentration and coagulability, that are promoted by hypoglycaemia could affect capillary blood flow and cause capillary closure, so exacerbating the pre-existing microangiopathy of diabetes.

Effects on quality of life

A major long-term psychological effect of recurrent hypoglycaemia is the impact that this can have on the everyday activities of people with diabetes and on their families. The manifestations of hypoglycaemia are unpleasant and frightening,[125] and the consequences of severe hypoglycaemia can be serious. Severe hypoglycaemia is very disruptive and can impinge on every aspect of daily life. It can occur at any time of the day or night and is frequently unpredictable. The ever-present risk of hypoglycaemia and its possible ramifications often causes long-term emotional distress. Psychological manifestations include decreased happiness, chronic anxiety and depression,[48,126] and, in a few extreme cases, a phobia develops.[127] Hypoglycaemia can therefore generate emotional upset,[126] difficulties with personal relationships and problems at school or at work.[48] Such is the fear of hypoglycaemia and its potential outcomes that many people with diabetes who have experienced multiple episodes of severe hypoglycaemia regard it with the same degree of worry as the development of long-term complications of diabetes such as sight-threatening retinopathy or renal failure (Figure 5.7).[60] Recurrent hypoglycaemia can therefore have significant psychological sequelae that affect the subsequent behaviour and the approach to self-management of diabetes. This can influence the approach to self-care of dia-

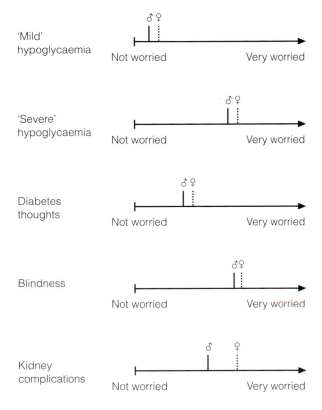

Figure 5.7

Results, on a visual analogue scale, showing attitudes towards different aspects of diabetes, as indicated by patients with Type 1 diabetes. Reproduced from Pramming et al.,[60] with the permission of Diabetic Medicine.

betes by the individual or by carers and relatives, and may encourage poor or suboptimal glycaemic control in an attempt to avoid severe hypo-glycaemia.[128] Hypoglycaemia may also cause significant psychological upset in family members, particularly of spouses or partners[129] and the parents of diabetic children,[130] and disrupt the everyday lives of close family and friends.

Insulin replacement therapy is a lifelong treatment for individuals with Type 1 diabetes and the problems (real and potential) associated with hypoglycaemia may necessitate considerable adjustments to daily lifestyle. Special precautions need to be taken and activities planned with care when embarking on physical exercise, recreational activities, travel and holidays. Hypoglycaemia is a potential hazard when driving,[131,132] and can affect employment prospects. Vocational driving licences are not permitted for drivers taking insulin and the development of impaired awareness of hypoglycaemia or recurrent severe hypoglycaemia can cause the revocation of an ordinary driving licence. Because hypoglycaemia is a potential risk in the workplace, insulin-treated diabetic patients are excluded from dangerous or high-risk occupations, and occasionally may suffer from discrimination by potential employers. The risk and development of hypoglycaemia at work can result in enforced changes in, and sometimes loss, of employment. In the longer term, all of these problems may enforce lifestyle changes. Recurrent hypoglycaemia may therefore cause profound physical and psychological morbidity, and the long-term burden of restrictions that may be imposed by the risk of hypoglycaemia is therefore considerable.

It is important that the long-term sequelae of recurrent hypoglycaemia are fully appreciated and addressed by diabetes specialists and other health-care professionals. It is evident that individual susceptibility to the detrimental effects of hypoglycaemia may vary. If individuals are experiencing recurrent severe hypoglycaemia with associated morbidity, their therapeutic goals for glycaemic control need to be modified. Suboptimal glycaemic control may have to be accepted for those who are at an increased risk of suffering severe hypoglycaemia and for individuals who appear to be more vulnerable to the deleterious effects of hypoglycaemia.

Conclusions

- Hypoglycaemia is a common side effect of insulin therapy in people with diabetes and can have important long-term consequences;
- isolated episodes of acute hypoglycaemia can cause coma, convulsions, neurological deficit, physical injury or acute vascular events, such as myocardial infarction or stroke, while repeated exposure to hypoglycaemia may cause more subtle long-term sequelae to affect cognitive function, impair intellectual ability and alter mood, which are less readily apparent;
- recurrent episodes of hypoglycaemia may promote the development of hypoglycaemia-associated syndromes, such as impaired awareness of hypoglycaemia, counterregulatory deficiencies and central autonomic failure, through effects on glycaemic thresholds for neuroendocrine and symptomatic responses to hypoglycaemia and with evidence of cerebral adaptation to low blood glucose concentrations;
- it has been surmised, on hypothetical grounds, that recurrent hypoglycaemia may aggravate existing microvascular disease by promoting capillary closure;
- frequent exposure to hypoglycaemia can significantly influence the quality of life of affected individuals and their relatives, and influence employment, driving, travel and recreation.

References

1. MacLeod KM, Hepburn DA, Frier BM. Frequency and morbidity of severe hypoglycaemia in insulin-treated diabetic patients. Diabet Med 1993; 10:238–45.

2. Diabetes Control and Complications Trial Research Group. The effect of intensive treatment of diabetes and the development and progression of long-term complications in insulin dependent diabetes mellitus. New Engl J Med 1993; 329:977–86.

3. Reichard P, Pihl M. Mortality and treatment side-effects during long-term intensified insulin treatment in the Stockholm Diabetes Intervention Study. Diabetes 1994; 43:313–17.

4. Hevener AL, Bergman RN, Donovan CM. Portal vein afferents are critical for the sympathoadrenal response to hypoglycemia. Diabetes 2000; 49:8–12.

5. Cryer PE, Fisher JN, Shamoon H. Hypoglycemia. Diabetes Care 1994; 17:734–55.

6. Mitrakou A, Ryan C, Veneman T, et al. Hierarchy of glycemic thresholds for counterregulatory hormone secretion, symptoms and cerebral dysfunction. Am J Physiol 1991; 266:E67–E74.

7. Fisher BM, Gillen G, Dargie, HJ, et al. The effects of insulin-induced hypoglycaemia on cardiovascular function in normal man: studies using radionuclide ventriculography. Diabetologia 1987; 30:841–5.

8. Fisher BM, Frier BM. Effect on vascular disease. In: Frier BM, Fisher BM, editors. Hypoglycaemia and diabetes: clinical and physiological aspects. London: Edward Arnold; 1993:355–61.

9. Tallroth G, Ryding E, Agardh C-D. Regional cerebral blood flow in normal man during insulin-induced hypoglycemia and in the recovery period following glucose infusion. Metabolism 1992; 41: 717–21.

10. Fisher BM, Quin JD, Rumley A, et al. Effects of acute insulin-induced hypoglycaemia on haemostasis, fibrinolysis and haemorrheology in insulin-dependent diabetic patients and control subjects. Clin Sci 1991; 80: 525–31.

11. Fisher BM, Heller SR. Mortality, cardiovascular morbidity and possible effects of hypoglycaemia on diabetic complications. In: Frier BM, Fisher BM, editors. Hypoglycaemia in clinical diabetes. Chichester: John Wiley and Sons; 1999:167–86.

12. Fisher BM, Thomson I, Hepburn DA, Frier BM. Effects of adrenergic blockade on serum potassium changes in response to acute insulin-induced hypoglycemia in non-diabetic humans. Diabetes Care 1991; 14:548–52.

13. Marques JLB, George E, Peacey SR, et al. Altered ventricular repolarisation during hypoglycaemia in patients with diabetes. Diabet Med 1997; 14:648–54.

14. Pladziewicz DS, Nesto RW. Hypoglycemia-induced silent myocardial ischemia. Am J Cardiol 1989; 63:1531–2.

15. Hepburn DA, Steel JM, Frier BM. Hypoglycemic convulsions cause serious musculo-skeletal injuries in patients with IDDM. Diabetes Care 1989; 12:32–4.

16. Pramming S, Thorsteinsson B, Theilgaard A, Pinner EM, Binder C. Cognitive function during hypoglycaemia in Type 1 diabetes mellitus. Br Med J 1986; 292: 647–50.

17. Deary IJ. Symptoms of hypoglycaemia and effects on mental

performance and emotion. In: Frier BM, Fisher BM, editors. Hypoglycaemia in clinical diabetes. Chichester: John Wiley and Sons; 1999:29–54.

18. Blackman JD, Towle VL, Sturis J, et al. Hypoglycemic thresholds for cognitive dysfunction in IDDM. Diabetes 1992; 41:392–9.

19. Lindgren M, Eckert B, Stenberg G, Agardh CD. Restitution of neurophysiological functions, performance and subjective symptoms after moderate insulin-induced hypoglycaemia in non-diabetic men. Diabet Med 1996; 13:218–25.

20. Strachan MWJ, Ewing FME, Deary IJ, Frier BM. Recovery of cognitive function and mood after severe hypoglycemia in insulin-treated diabetes mellitus. Diabetes Care 2000; 23:305–12.

21. Pramming S, Thorsteinsson B, Stigsby B, Binder C. Glycaemic threshold for changes in electroencephalograms during hypoglycaemia in patients with insulin dependent diabetes. Br Med J 1988; 296:665–7.

22. Tribl G, Howorka K, Heger G, et al. EEG topography during insulin-induced hypoglycemia in patients with insulin-dependent diabetes mellitus. Eur Neurol 1996; 36: 303–9.

23. Bjorgaas M, Sand T, Vik T, Jorde R. Quantitative EEG during controlled hypoglycaemia in diabetic and non-diabetic children. Diabet Med 1998; 15:30–7.

24. Perros P, Deary IJ. Long-term effects of hypoglycaemia on cognitive function and the brain in diabetes. In: Frier BM, Fisher BM, editors. Hypoglycaemia in clinical diabetes. Chichester: John Wiley and Sons; 1999:187–210.

25. Critchley JAJH, Proudfoot AT, Boyd SG, et al. Deaths and paradoxes after intentional insulin overdosage. Br Med J 1984; 289:225.

26. Arky RA, Veverbrants E, Abramson EA. Irreversible hypoglycemia. A complication of alcohol and insulin. J Am Med Ass 1968; 206:575–8.

27. Agardh C-D, Rosen I, Ryding E. Persistent vegetative state with high cerebral blood flow following profound hypoglycemia. Ann Neurol 1983; 14:482–6.

28. Cotman CW, Iversen LL. Excitatory amino acids in the brain focus on NMDA receptors. Trends Neurosci 1987; 10:263–5.

29. Choi DW. Methods for antagonising glutamate neurotoxicity. Cerebrovasc Brain Metab Rev 1990; 2:105–47.

30. Auer RN, Wieloch T, Olsson Y, Siesjo BK. The distribution of hypoglycaemic brain damage. Acta Neuropath 1984; 64: 177–91.

31. Patrick AW, Campbell IW. Fatal hypoglycaemia in insulin-treated diabetes mellitus: clinical features and neuropathological consequences. Diabet Med 1990; 7: 349–54.

32. Chalmers JC, Risk MTA, Kean DM, et al. Severe amnesia after hypoglycemia. Clinical, psychometric, and magnetic resonance imaging correlations. Diabetes Care 1991; 14:922–5.

33. Perros P, Sellar RJ, Frier BM. Chronic pontine dysfunction following insulin-induced hypoglycemia in an IDDM patient. Diabetes Care 1994; 17:725–7.

34. Tattersall RB, Gale EAM. Mortality. In: Frier BM, Fisher BM, editors. Hypoglycaemia and diabetes: clinical and physiological aspects. London: Edward Arnold; 1993:191–8.

35. Laing SP, Swerdlow AJ, Slater SD, et al. The British Diabetic Association Cohort Study, II: cause-specific mortality in patients with insulin-treated dia-

betes mellitus. Diabet Med 1999; 16:466–71.

36. Campbell I. Dead in bed syndrome: a new manifestation of nocturnal hypoglycaemia? Diabet Med 1991; 8:3–4.

37. Tattersall RB, Gill GV. Unexpected deaths of Type 1 diabetic patients. Diabet Med 1991; 8:49–58.

38. Sartor G, Dahlquist G. Short-term mortality in childhood onset insulin-dependent diabetes mellitus: a high frequency of unexpected deaths in bed. Diabet Med 1995; 12:607–11.

39. Thordarson H, Sovik O. Dead in bed syndrome in young diabetic patients in Norway. Diabet Med 1995; 12:782–7.

40. Lawrence IJ, Weston PJ, Bennet MA, et al. Is impaired baroreflex sensitivity a predictor or cause of sudden death in insulin dependent diabetes mellitus? Diabet Med 1997; 14:82–5.

41. Weston PJ, Gill GV. Is undetected autonomic dysfunction responsible for sudden death in Type 1 diabetes mellitus? The 'dead in bed' syndrome revisited. Diabet Med 1999; 16:626–31.

42. Ryan CM. Neuropsychological complications of Type 1 diabetes. Diabetes Care 1988; 11:86–93.

43. Dejgaard A, Gade A, Larsson H, et al. Evidence for diabetic encephalopathy. Diabet Med 1991; 8:162–7.

44. McCall AL. The impact of diabetes on the CNS. Diabetes 1992; 41:557–70.

45. Deary IJ. The effects of diabetes on cognitive function. In: Marshall SM, Home PD, Rizza RA, editors. Diabetes annual. Amsterdam: Elsevier Science BV; 1998: 97–118.

46. Biessels GJ, Kappelle AC, Bravenboer B, et al. Cerebral function in diabetes mellitus. Diabetologia 1994; 37: 643–50.

47. Snook JA, Vanderstar R, Weller RO. Insulinoma producing progressive neurological deterioration over 30 years. Br Med J 1986; 293:241–2.

48. Gold AE, Deary IJ, Jones RW, et al. Severe deterioration in cognitive function and personality in five patients with long-standing diabetes: a complication of diabetes or a consequence of treatment? Diabet Med 1994; 11: 499–505.

49. Rovet JF, Ehrlich RM, Hoppe M. Intellectual deficits associated with early onset of insulin-dependent diabetes mellitus in children. Diabetes Care 1987; 10:510–15.

50. Golden MP, Ingersol GM, Brack CJ, et al. Longitudinal relationship of asymptomatic hypoglycemia to cognitive function in IDDM. Diabetes Care 1989; 12: 89–93.

51. Bjørgass M, Gimse R, Vik T, Sand T. Cognitive function in Type 1 diabetic children with and without episodes of severe hypoglycaemia. Paediatr 1997; 86: 148–53.

52. Ryan CM. Effects of diabetes mellitus on neurophysiological functioning: a lifespan perspective. Seminars Clin Neuropsychiat 1997; 2:4–14.

53. Northam EA, Anderson PJ, Werther GA, et al. Neuropsychological complications of IDDM in children 2 years after disease onset. Diabetes Care 1998; 21: 379–84.

54. Northam EA, Anderson PJ, Werther G, et al. Neuropsychological profiles of children with Type 1 diabetes 6 years after disease onset. Diabetes Care 2001; 24:1541–6.

55. Ryan CM, Vega A, Longstreet C, Drash A. Neuropsychological changes in adolescents with

insulin-dependent diabetes. J Consult Clin Psychol 1984; 52:335–42.

56. Rovet J, Alvarez M. Attentional functioning in children and adolescents with IDDM. Diabetes Care 1997; 20:803–10.

57. The Diabetes Control and Complications Trial Research Group. Effects of intensive diabetes therapy on neuropsychological function in adults in the Diabetes Control and Complications Trial. Ann Intern Med 1996; 124: 379–88.

58. Reichard P, Pihl M, Rosenqvist U, Sule J. Complications in IDDM are caused by elevated blood glucose level: the Stockholm Diabetes Intervention Study (SDIS) at 10-year follow up. Diabetologia 1996; 39:1483–8.

59. Austin EJ, Deary IJ. Effects of repeated hypoglycemia on cognitive function: a psychometrically validated reanalysis of the Diabetes Control and Complications Trial data. Diabetes Care 1999; 22:1273–7.

60. Pramming S, Thorsteinsson B, Bendtson I, Binder C. Symptomatic hypoglycaemia in 411 Type 1 diabetic patients. Diabet Med 1991; 8:217–22.

61. Bale RN. Brain damage in diabetes mellitus. Br J Psychol 1973; 122:337–41.

62. Skenazy JA, Bigler ED. Neuropsychological findings in diabetes mellitus. J Clin Psychol 1984; 40:246–50.

63. Wredling R, Levander S, Adamson U, Lins PE. Permanent neuropsychological impairment after recurrent episodes of severe hypoglycaemia in man. Diabetologia 1990; 33:152–7.

64. Langan SJ, Deary IJ, Hepburn DA, Frier BM. Cumulative cognitive impairment following recurrent severe hypoglycaemia in adult patients with insulin-treated diabetes mellitus. Diabetologia 1991; 34:337–44.

65. Deary IJ, Crawford JR, Hepburn DA, et al. Severe hypoglycemia and intelligence in adult patients with insulin-treated diabetes. Diabetes 1993; 42:341–4.

66. Deary IJ, Langan SJ, Graham KS, et al. Recurrent severe hypoglycaemia, intelligence, and speed of information processing. Intelligence 1992; 16:337–59.

67. Lincoln NB, Kirk BA, Faleiro RM, et al. Effect of long-term glycemic control on cognitive function. Diabetes Care 1996; 19:656–8.

68. Hepburn DA, Patrick AW, Brash HM, et al. Hypoglycaemia unawareness in Type 1 diabetes: a lower plasma glucose is required to stimulate sympathoadrenal activation. Diabet Med 1991; 8:934–45.

69. Gold AE, MacLeod KM, Deary IJ, Frier BM. Hypoglycemia-induced cognitive dysfunction in diabetes mellitus: effect of hypoglycemia unawareness. Physiol Behav 1995; 58:501–11.

70. MacLeod KM, Deary IJ, Graham KS, et al. Hypoglycaemia unawareness in adult patients with Type 1 diabetes: relationship to severe hypoglycaemia and cognitive impairment. Diabet Nutr Metab 1994; 7: 205–12.

71. Araki Y, Nomura M, Tanaka H, et al. MRI of the brain in diabetes mellitus. Neuroradiology 1994; 36:101–3.

72. Pantoni L, Garcia JH. The significance of cerebral white matter abnormalities 100 years after Binswanger's report. Stroke 1996; 26:1293–301.

73. Awad IA, Johnson PC, Spetzler RF, Hodak JA. Incidental sub-cortical lesions identified on magnetic resonance imaging in the elderly, II: post-mortem pathologi-

cal correlations. Stroke 1986; 17: 1090–7.

74. Lunetta M, Damanti AR, Fabbri G, et al. Evidence by magnetic resonance imaging of cerebral alterations of atrophy type in young insulin-dependent diabetic patients. J Endocr Invest 1994; 17:241–5.

75. Perros P, Deary IJ, Sellar RJ, et al. Brain abnormalities demonstrated by magnetic resonance imaging in adult IDDM patients with and without a history of recurrent severe hypoglycemia. Diabetes Care 1997; 20:1013–18.

76. Junque C, Pujol J, Vendrell P, et al. Leukoaraiosis on magnetic resonance imaging and speed of mental processing. Archs Neurol 1990; 47:151–6.

77. Garde E, Mortensen EL, Krabbe K, et al. Relation between age-related decline in intelligence and cerebral white matter hyperintensities in healthy octogenerians: a longitudinal study. Lancet 2000; 356:628–34.

78. deGroot JC, deLeeuw FE, Oudkerk M, et al. Cerebral white matter lesions and cognitive function: the Rotterdam Scan Study. Ann Neurol 2000; 47:145–51.

79. Ferguson SC, McCrimmon RJ, Perros P, et al. Severe hypoglycaemia, cognition and MRI structural abnormalities in young patients with Type 1 diabetes. Diabetologia 1999; 42(Suppl 1): A72 (abstract).

80. Ryan CM, Williams TM, Finegold DN, Orchard TJ. Cognitive dysfunction in adults with type 1 (insulin-dependent) diabetes mellitus of long duration: effects of recurrent hypoglycaemia and other chronic complications. Diabetologia 1993; 36:329–34.

81. Hepburn DA, Patrick AW, Eadington DW, et al. Unawareness of hypoglycaemia in insulin-treated diabetic patients: prevalence and relationship to autonomic neuropathy. Diabet Med 1990; 7:711–17.

82. Gerich JE, Mokan M, Veneman T, et al. Hypoglycemia unawareness. Endocr Rev 1991; 12: 356–71.

83. Gold AE, MacLeod KM, Frier BM. Frequency of hypoglycemia in patients with type 1 diabetes with impaired awareness of hypoglycemia. Diabetes Care 1994; 17:697–703.

84. Mokan M, Mitrakou A, Veneman T, et al. Hypoglycemia unawareness in IDDM. Diabetes Care 1994; 17:1397–403.

85. Gerich JE, Langlois M, Noacco C, et al. Lack of glucagon response to hypoglycemia in diabetes: evidence for an intrinsic pancreatic alpha cell defect. Science 1973; 182: 171–3.

86. Bolli G, De Feo P, Compagnucci P, et al. Abnormal glucose counterregulation in insulin-dependent diabetes mellitus. Interaction of anti-insulin antibodies and impaired glucagon and epinephrine secretion. Diabetes 1983; 32:134–41.

87. Hirsch BR, Shamoon H. Defective epinephrine and growth hormone responses in Type 1 diabetes are stimulus specific. Diabetes 1987; 36:20–6.

88. Frier BM, Fisher BM, Gray CE, Beastall GH. Counterregulatory hormonal responses in Type 1 (insulin-dependent) diabetes: evidence for diminished hypothalamic–pituitary hormonal secretion. Diabetologia 1988; 31:421–9.

89. Kinsley BT, Widom B, Utzschneider K, Simonson DC. Stimulus specificity of defects in counterregulatory hormone secretion in insulin-dependent diabetes mellitus: effect of glycemic control. J

Clin Endocr Metab 1994; 79: 1383–9.

90. White NH, Skor DA, Cryer PE, et al. Identification of type 1 diabetic patients at increased risk for hypoglycemia during intensive therapy. New Engl J Med 1983; 308:485–91.

91. Gerich JE, Bolli GB. Counterregulatory failure. In: Frier BM, Fisher BM, editors. Hypoglycaemia and diabetes: clinical and physiological aspects. London: Edward Arnold; 1993:253–67.

92. Dagogo-Jack SE, Craft S, Cryer PE. Hypoglycemia-associated autonomic failure in insulin dependent diabetes mellitus. J Clin Invest 1993; 91:819–28.

93. Amiel SA, Sherwin RS, Simonson DC, Tamborlane WV. Effect of intensive insulin therapy on glycemic thresholds for counterregulatory hormone release. Diabetes 1988; 37:901–7.

94. Amiel SA, Tamborlane WV, Simonson DC, Sherwin RS. Defective glucose counterregulation after strict glycemic control of insulin-dependent diabetes mellitus. New Engl J Med 1987; 316:1376–83.

95. Widom B, Simonson DC. Glycemic control and neuropsychologic function during hypoglycemia in patients with insulin-dependent diabetes mellitus. Ann Intern Med 1990; 112: 904–12.

96. Boyle PJ, Nagy RJ, O'Connor AM, et al. Adaptation in brain glucose uptake following recurrent hypoglycemia. Proc Natl Acad Sci USA 1994; 91:9352–6.

97. Boyle PJ, Kempers SF, O'Connor AM, Nagy RJ. Brain glucose uptake and unawareness of hypoglycemia in patients with insulin-dependent diabetes mellitus. New Engl J Med 1995; 333:

1726–31.

98. Kinsley BT, Widom B, Simonson DC. Differential regulation of counterregulatory hormone secretion and symptoms during hypoglycemia in IDDM. Effect of glycemic control. Diabetes Care 1995; 18:17–26.

99. Spyer G, Hattersley AT, Macdonald IA, et al. Hypoglycaemic counter-regulation at normal blood glucose concentrations in patients with well controlled Type 2 diabetes. Lancet 2000; 356: 1970–4.

100. Ziegler D, Hubinger A, Muhlen H, Gries FA. Effects of previous glycaemic control on the onset and magnitude of cognitive dysfunction during hypoglycaemia in Type 1 (insulin-dependent) diabetic patients. Diabetologia 1992; 35: 828–34.

101. Veneman T, Mitrakou A, Mokan M, et al. Induction of hypoglycemia unawareness by asymptomatic nocturnal hypoglycemia. Diabetes 1993; 42: 1233–7.

102. Jones TW, Borg WP, Borg MA, et al. Resistance to neuroglycopenia: an adaptive response during intensive insulin treatment of diabetes. J Clin Endocr Med 1997; 82:1713–18.

103. Ovalle F, Fanelli CG, Paramore DS, et al. Brief twice weekly episodes of hypoglycemia reduce detection of clinical hypoglycemia in Type 1 diabetes mellitus. Diabetes 1998; 47:1472–9.

104. Fanelli CG, Paramore DS, Hershey T, et al. Impact of nocturnal hypoglycemia on hypoglycemic cognitive dysfunction in Type 1 diabetes. Diabetes 1998; 47: 1920–7.

105. Taverna MJ, M'Bemba J, Sola A, et al. Insufficient adaptation of hypoglycaemia threshold for cognitive impairment in tightly con-

trolled Type 1 diabetes. Diabete Metab (Paris) 2000; 26:58–64.

106. Amiel SA, Pottinger RC, Archibald HR, et al. Effect of antecedent glucose control on cerebral function during hypoglycemia. Diabetes Care 1991; 14:109–18.

107. Maran A, Lomas J, Macdonald IA, Amiel SA. Lack of preservation of higher brain function during hypoglycaemia in patients with intensively-treated IDDM. Diabetologia 1995; 38:1412–18.

108. Hvidberg A, Fanelli CG, Hershey T, et al. Impact of recent antecedent hypoglycemia on hypoglycemic cognitive dysfunction in non-diabetic humans. Diabetes 1996; 45:1030–6.

109. Amiel SA. Cognitive function testing in studies of acute hypoglycaemia: rights and wrongs? Diabetologia 1998; 41:713–19.

110. Fanelli CG, Pampanelli S, Porcellati F, Bolli GB. Shift of glycaemic thresholds for cognitive function in hypoglycaemia unawareness in humans. Diabetologia 1998; 41: 720–3.

111. Heller SR, Cryer PE. Reduced neuroendocrine and symptomatic responses to subsequent hypoglycemia after 1 episode of hypoglycemia in nondiabetic humans. Diabetes 1991; 40:223–6.

112. Davis MR, Mellman M, Shamoon H. Further defects in counterregulatory responses induced by recurrent hypoglycemia in IDDM. Diabetes 1992; 41:1335–40.

113. MacLeod KM, Hepburn DA, Deary IJ, et al. Regional cerebral blood flow in IDDM patients: effects of diabetes and of recurrent severe hypoglycaemia. Diabetologia 1994; 37:257–63.

114. MacLeod KM, Gold AE, Ebmeier KP, et al. The effects of hypoglycemia on relative cerebral blood flow distribution in patients with Type 1 (insulin-dependent)

diabetes and impaired hypoglycemia awareness. Metabolism 1996; 45:974–80.

115. Cryer PE. Iatrogenic hypoglycemia as a cause of hypoglycemia-associated autonomic failure in IDDM. A vicious circle. Diabetes 1992; 41:255–60.

116. Cranston I, Lomas J, Maran A, et al. Restoration of hypoglycaemia awareness in patients with long-duration insulin-dependent diabetes. Lancet 1994; 344: 283–7.

117. Dagogo-Jack S, Rattarasarn C, Cryer PE. Reversal of hypoglycemia unawareness, but not defective glucose counterregulation, in IDDM. Diabetes 1994; 43: 1426–34.

118. Fanelli CG, Epifano L, Rambotti AM, et al. Meticulous prevention of hypoglycemia normalizes the glycemic thresholds and magnitude of most of neuroendocrine responses to, symptoms of, and cognitive function during hypoglycemia in intensively treated patients with short-term IDDM. Diabetes 1993; 42:1683–9.

119. Frier BM, Hilsted J. Does hypoglycaemia aggravate the complications of diabetes? Lancet 1985; 326:1175–7.

120. Hanssen KF, Dahl-Jorgensen K, Lauritzen T, et al. Diabetic control and microvascular complications: the near normoglycaemic experience. Diabetologia 1986; 29: 677–84.

121. Kohner EM, McLeod D, Marshall J. Diabetic eye disease. In: Keen H, Jarrett J, editors. Complications of diabetes, 2nd edition. London: Edward Arnold; 1975: 62–82.

122. Tasman W. Diabetic vitreous haemorrhage and its relationship to hypoglycemia. Mod Probl Ophthal 1974; 20:413–14.

123. Frier BM, Hepburn DA, Fisher BM, Barrie T. Fall in intraocular

pressure during acute hypogly-caemia in patients with insulin-dependent diabetes. Br Med J 1987; 294:610–11.

124. Patrick AW, Hepburn DA, Swainson CP, Frier BM. Changes in renal function during insulin-induced hypoglycaemia in Type 1 diabetes. Diabet Med 1992; 9: 150–5.

125. Sanders K, Mills J, Martin FIR, Horne DJD. Emotional attitudes in adult insulin-dependent diabetics. J Psychosom Res 1975; 19: 241–6.

126. Wredling RAM, Theorell PGT, Roll HM, et al. Psychosocial state of patients with IDDM prone to recurrent episodes of severe hypoglycemia. Diabetes Care 1992; 15:518–21.

127. Gold AE, Deary IJ, Frier BM. Hypoglycaemia and non-cognitive aspects of psychological function in insulin-dependent (Type 1) diabetes mellitus (IDDM). Diabet Med 1997; 14:111–18.

128. Thompson CJ, Cummings JFR, Chalmers J, et al. How have patients reacted to the implications of the DCCT? Diabetes Care 1996; 19:876–8.

129. Gonder-Frederick L, Cox D, Kovatchev B, et al. The psychosocial impact of severe hypoglycemic episodes on spouses of patients with IDDM. Diabetes Care 1997; 20: 1543–6.

130. Clarke WL, Gonder-Frederick LA, Miller S, et al. Maternal fear of hypoglycemia in their children with insulin-dependent diabetes mellitus. J Pediat Endocr Metab 1998; 4:189–94.

131. Eadington DW, Frier BM. Type 1 diabetes and driving experience: an 8 year cohort study. Diabet Med 1989; 6:137–41.

132. Cox DJ, Gonder-Frederick LA, Kovatchev BP, et al. Progressive hypoglycemia's impact on driving simulation performance: occurrence, awareness and correction. Diabetes Care 2000; 23: 163–70.

6
What is the role of the thiazolidinediones (glitazones) in clinical practice?

Elaine Murphy and John J Nolan

Introduction

Type 2 diabetes is a chronic, progressive, metabolic disorder character-ized by defects in both insulin action and insulin secretion.[1-5] Debate continues about whether insulin resistance or impaired insulin secretion is the primary initiating event, although both are clearly implicated in the development of overt diabetes. In patients with established Type 2 dia-betes, basal hepatic glucose output is increased, insulin-stimulated mus-cle glucose uptake is markedly reduced and, despite circulating hyperinsulinaemia, the beta cell response to hyperglycaemia is inade-quate in absolute terms.[5]

The thiazolidinediones (often referred to as glitazones) are the first of a new generation of oral antidiabetic agents that, in addition to their hypo-glycaemic properties, have been shown to improve insulin action in ani-mal models of obesity and Type 2 diabetes as well as Type 2 diabetes and pre-diabetic conditions in humans (Figure 6.1).[6-19] Their clinical development and the first years of their application to clinical practice have coincided with a period of rapid acceleration in the prevalence of Type 2 diabetes throughout the world and a relatively sudden change in the age of presentation of this disease, with a shift towards younger age at onset and an emerging epidemic of disease developing in children, adolescents and young adults.[20,21] The glitazones have begun to be used clinically just as the findings from the landmark UK Prospective Diabetes Study (UKPDS) have been published. The UKPDS has clearly demonstrated that better glycaemic control in Type 2 diabetes is directly translated to a reduction in microvascular (glucose-related) complica-tions.[22] Current consensus for treatment is that the long-term goal should be near-normal glycaemia in the majority of patients. Unfortunately, the UKPDS has also shown that sustained glycemic control was not possible beyond the initial 3–5 years after diagnosis during treatment with lifestyle changes, sulphonylureas, metformin and insulin (Figure 6.2).[23] Loss of insulin secretion and loss of peripheral insulin sensitivity are the key to

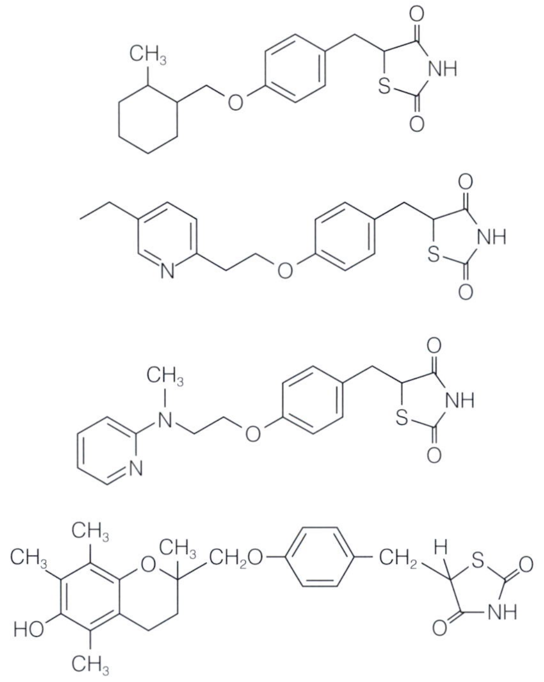

Ciglitazone

Pioglitazone

Rosiglitazone

Troglitazone

Figure 6.1

Structures of the thiazolidinediones. Ciglitazone, the first of the thiazolidinediones, did not reach clinical development. Troglitazone has been withdrawn from the market because of reports of hepatotoxicity. Rosiglitazone and pioglitazone are licensed for use as oral combination therapy in patients with Type 2 diabetes.

this inexorable deterioration in glycaemic control, despite treatment with conventional agents.

In addition, the UKPDS has demonstrated that the prevention of macrovascular disease in Type 2 diabetes, particularly coronary artery disease and stroke, is more difficult than controlling microvascular disease alone. The glitazone era (or the post-UKPDS era) coincides with a period of better understanding of the mechanisms by which Type 2 diabetes is associated with increased risk of atherosclerotic vascular disease. It is now clear that hyperglycaemia is not the only metabolic manifestation of Type 2 diabetes. These patients almost always have a complex high-risk cardiovascular syndrome that includes obesity, hypertension, dyslipidaemia, defects of thrombosis and fibrinolysis, and accelerated atherosclerosis.[5] Much evidence links the macrovascular risk factors and complications of Type 2 diabetes to insulin resistance, typical of the majority of subjects with this disease.[24,25] Among the established

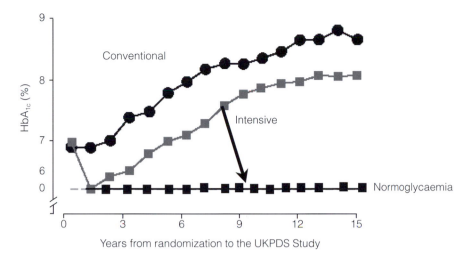

Figure 6.2

Long-term glycemic control in the intensively treated group compared with the conventionally treated group and long-term normoglycemia. [Adapted from UKPDS Study.[22]]

treatments for diabetes, only metformin has any effect on insulin resistance per se. This is likely to explain the slightly better macrovascular outcomes for metformin-treated subjects in the UKPDS group.[26,27] Prospective studies with cardiovascular end-points, such as the various lipid-lowering trials and the recent Heart Outcomes Prevention Evaluation (HOPE) and Microalbuminuria Cardiovascular, and Renal Outcomes in HOPE (Micro-HOPE) studies, have shown that subjects with Type 2 diabetes stand to benefit hugely from interventions that target their cardiovascular risk factors specifically.[28–32]

The thiazolidinediones have been the subject of several previous reviews.[10–12] Rosiglitazone (Avandia) and pioglitazone (Actos) are currently licensed for use in the UK. This review will therefore concentrate on current clinical practice and the more recently published literature on rosiglitazone and pioglitazone, summarizing their effects on glycaemic control and other markers of the metabolic syndrome, including hypertension, atherogenic lipid profile, obesity, circulating insulin and free fatty acid levels. The current and potential future role of these drugs in the treatment of Type 2 diabetes will be discussed. The evidence for a role for this class of drugs in pre-diabetes and in the metabolic syndrome generally will also be reviewed.

Despite a positive clinical development history, the glitazones have had a difficult phase of incorporation into clinical practice. Troglitazone, the first of the class to be licensed, was withdrawn from both the UK and US markets because of idiosyncratic and occasionally fatal hepatotoxicity.[33] The licensing authorities have been cautious with the successor drugs and the current licences for rosiglitazone and pioglitazone are restricted to combination therapy with sulphonylurea or metformin, and only where patients would not be suited to the sulphonlyurea–metformin combination first.[34,35] Monotherapy and combination with insulin is not licensed in Europe to date. These restrictions have been a major limitation for the glitazones, effectively precluding their use in the exact clinical settings in which they may offer most benefit.

Current guidelines for use

Recent guidelines (March 2001) from the National Institute for Clinical Excellence (NICE) state that rosiglitazone and pioglitazone may be regarded as alternatives.[35] Their use should be confined to those patients inadequately controlled on oral monotherapy and who are unable to tolerate, or have contraindications to, conventional combination therapy of metformin and a sulphonylurea. Neither drug should be used in patients with a history of cardiac failure, hepatic impairment or severe renal insufficiency. It is currently recommended that patients should have liver function tests prior to initiation of treatment, every 2 months for the first year and periodically thereafter. The need for further research to establish the long-term impact of these agents on cardiovascular risk factors, vascular complications and quality of life is acknowledged.

These guidelines and licensing restrictions seriously limit the current clinical use of the glitazones. The clinical development programme, along with several focused mechanistic studies, have clearly shown an advantage for the glitazones in drug-naïve subjects.[15,36,37] The same research has very clearly shown the complementary effects of the three major classes of oral antidiabetic drugs (sulphonylureas, metformin and glitazones) (Figure 6.3). Their effects are almost entirely synergistic and these agents are particularly effective in combination therapy.[38–44] Furthermore, the combination of glitazones with insulin is also a logical and very effective glucose-lowering strategy.[45–49] Insulin combination therapy is however not permitted. Current guidelines have unfortunately made even oral combination therapy a difficult option: in fact, patients with diabetes have to fail the combination of sulphonylurea and metformin before a glitazone can be introduced. The only exception would be the minority of patients for whom either sulphonlylurea or metformin is contraindicated. The difficulty with these regulations is that the glitazones can be deployed only under disadvantageous conditions, mainly to substitute one of the conventional oral agents after withdrawal. In most cases, this is likely to be of no net glycaemic benefit, since the glitazones are of similar glucose-lowering efficacy to the other two classes of drug. Withdrawal

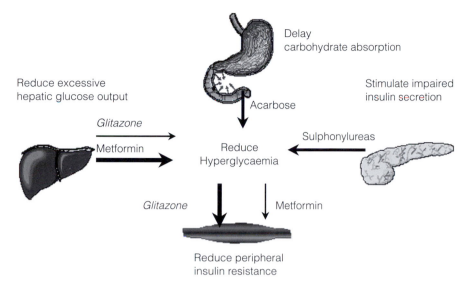

Figure 6.3
Complementary effects of oral hypoglycaemic agents.

of either sulphonylurea or metformin therapy will lead to a deterioration in glycaemic control, which at best might be restored to the previous baseline level by an appropriate dose of a glitazone. Triple combination therapy is not licensed and has not been the subject of any substantial research to date.

Perhaps a more important consideration is the range of additional effects the glitazones have been shown to have on those cardiovascular risk factors that are closely associated with insulin resistance. Their effects on insulin sensitivity far exceed the effects of any previous agent, including metformin.[50] A wide range of potentially beneficial effects has been shown on blood pressure, plasma lipoproteins, endothelial factors and urine albumin excretion.[51-60] This expanded non-glucose profile of the glitazones has raised expectations that these drugs may offer real additional benefit to patients in the long-term prevention of atherosclerotic cardiovascular disease. Testing this hypothesis will take at least several years and will need to be the subject of well-designed prospective trials. Such trials are now in the early stages of design or implementation. In summary, although there is a clear and logical role for the glitazones, even on glucose-lowering grounds alone, the current licensing restrictions and guidelines seriously limit the development of their potential role (Table 6.1).

Table 6.1 Thiazolidinediones – outstanding questions and controversies.

Exact molecular and physiological mechanisms of action?
Long-term efficacy in sustaining glycaemic control?
Long-term safety?
Role for early intervention in pre-diabetic conditions?
Role in the prevention of the macrovascular complications?
Licensing restrictions
Within-class variability (weight gain, lipids and adverse events)?

Mechanism of action

At present, neither the primary site of action nor the cellular mechanism of the thiazolidinediones is fully understood. They appear to exert their effects by altering the transcription of genes involved in carbohydrate and fat metabolism.[61–65] The thiazolidinediones are known to be ligands for the peroxisome proliferator-activated nuclear receptor-γ (PPARγ).[66,67] The usual physiological role of PPARγ is not yet clear. Within the nucleus, PPARγ exists as a heterodimer with another nuclear receptor, retinoid X (RXR). It appears that, upon ligand binding, a conformational change occurs in the PPARγ–RXR receptor complex. This conformational change alters the binding of local co-repressor/co-activator complexes, resulting in the binding of the complex to gene-promoter regions called PPAR response elements (PPRE) and the subsequent transcription of PPAR responsive genes (Figure 6.4).[68–71]

PPARγ is found in low concentrations in many tissues, including classical sites of insulin resistance, e.g. skeletal muscle and the liver, but it is within the adipocyte that the thiazolidinediones have been thought to exert their main effects.[72] Individuals with Type 2 diabetes have larger, more insulin-resistant adipocytes that produce higher circulating concentrations of free fatty acids (FFA). Raised FFA levels are associated with insulin resistance in peripheral tissues and with circulating hyperinsulinaemia.[73–74] The thiazolidinediones have been shown to reduce FFA and, consequently, to improve insulin sensitivity.[37] However, a recent report demonstrating that thiazolidinediones may have effects on normalizing lipid metabolism but not glucose metabolism, even in lipoatrophic (fat-free) diabetic mice, suggests that there may be an important direct action of the thiazolidinediones on other tissues, probably skeletal muscle, but that some additional signal is required from adipose tissue to skeletal muscle to improve glucose tolerance.[76,77]

An exciting new report establishes a link between thiazolidinedione action, an adipocyte gene, obesity and improvements in insulin sensitivity.[78] A novel adipocyte-specific gene, coding for a hormone, resistin, is downregulated by the thiazolidinediones, leading to reduced serum con-

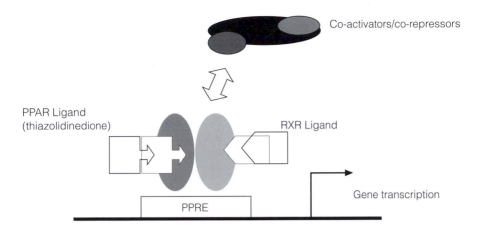

Co-activators/co-repressors

PPAR Ligand
(thiazolidinedione)

RXR Ligand

Gene transcription

PPRE

Figure 6.4
Mechanism of action of the thiazolidinediones. PPAR, proliferator-activated nuclear receptor; PPRE, peroxisome proliferator response element; RXR, retinoid X receptor.

centrations in vivo and reduced cellular expression in vitro. Resistin has been shown to be elevated in obese and diabetic mice, leading to impaired glucose tolerance in vivo. Therefore, resistin is an adipocyte-derived protein that contributes to insulin resistance in vivo and, as a putative hormone, may have effects on other insulin-responsive tissues as a modulator of the insulin-signalling pathway.[79]

Rosiglitazone

Published data are currently available from the clinical development programme in which more than 5000 patients with Type 2 diabetes have been treated with rosiglitazone alone or in combination with other antidiabetic agents. Rosiglitazone has a higher binding affinity for PPAR than either troglitazone or pioglitazone and is the most potent of the licensed thiazolidinediones. In controlled clinical trials with rosiglitazone monotherapy other oral agents were withdrawn 3–4 weeks before randomization to rosiglitazone 0.1–12mg daily, given either singly or in divided doses, or placebo.[14,36,37,80,81] Study duration varied from 8 to 52 weeks, with additional long-term (4 year) extension studies already underway.[82] A dose-dependent reduction in fasting plasma glucose (FPG) (−9 to −19% from baseline) and glycated haemoglobin HbA_{1c}

was seen with a daily dose of rosiglitazone of 4–8mg. No additional gly-caemic benefit was gained with a daily dose of 12mg.[80,81] 4mg per day, with a once daily dosing, is therapeutically equivalent to rosiglitazone given in divided doses, while at 8mg per day, twice daily administration (i.e. 4mg bd) is clearly more effective. Treatment effect is noticeable by weeks 2–4, reaches a maximum effect by weeks 8–12, with beneficial effects maintained for up to 1 year.[36,37] Drug-naïve patients show a better response to therapy than those previously treated with other agents, either alone or in combination.[37]

Statistically significant dose-related reductions in circulating FFA levels (-15 to -32% reduction from baseline) are seen with rosiglitazone given at doses of 8–12mg daily.[37,80,81] This effect is not consistent at doses of 4mg daily.[37,81]

More prolonged treatment with rosiglitazone (and the other glitazones – see below) has been shown to lead to weight gain of the order of 1–3%, or 1–5kg typically.[37,80,81] This weight gain, although undesirable, occurs without a change in the waist-to-hip ratio (where this has been measured) and may reflect either thiazolidinedione-related fluid retention or subcuta-neous fat accumulation, both of which confer a lower cardiovascular risk than accumulation of intra-abdominal adiposity. Alterations in body fat distribution, with resultant increases in subcutaneous fat mass, have already been confirmed in patients taking troglitazone.[83,84] The long-term significance of these alterations in body weight and fat distribution remain to be established by prospective studies and clinical experience, and are likely to continue to remain somewhat controversial until they are better understood.

Rosiglitazone has also been evaluated in combination therapy with sulphonylureas, metformin or insulin in randomized, placebo-controlled trials. In a head-to-head study over 52 weeks, in which glibenclamide was optimally titrated over the first 12 weeks, although the initial response was better with glibenclamide, rosiglitazone at 8mg daily was more effec-tive in maintaining reductions in FPG.[85] End-point HbA$_{1c}$ levels were com-parable between the two groups after 1 year of treatment. However, FPG and HbA$_{1c}$ were beginning to rise in the glibenclamide-treated group at 38 weeks, in contrast to a stable plateau in the rosiglitazone-treated group. Rosiglitazone, 2 or 4mg (in divided doses), when added to sulphonylurea treatment produced a significant dose-related reduction in both FPG and HbA$_{1c}$ after 26 weeks (-8 to -18% from baseline and -5 to -10% from baseline, respectively).[38] The improvement in HbA$_{1c}$ was similar for all sulphonlyurea drugs tested – gliclazide, glibenclamide and glipizide – and contrasts with a 2% increase in HbA$_{1c}$ in patients who continued on treatment with a sulphonylurea alone.

The addition of an insulin-sensitizer agent, such as rosiglitazone to metformin, rather than to an insulin secretagogue may be a more rational approach to the treatment of insulin-resistant patients with Type 2 diabetes. In a 26-week study, rosiglitazone (4 or 8mg daily) added to the treatment of patients inadequately controlled near-maximal metformin (2.5g daily), producing additional dose-related reductions in FPG and HbA$_{1c}$ of -15 to -22% and -6 to -9% from baseline, respectively.[39] This effect was seen across a range of body mass indices (BMI) ($< 25->$ 30kgm^{-2}) but was most pronounced in the more obese patients.[40] The reduction in HbA$_{1c}$ was sustained in patients treated with 8mg of rosiglitazone in addition to 2.5mg of metformin over a 24-month open-labelled extension study.[41] In 319 patients with Type 2 diabetes, poorly controlled on insulin (HbA$_{1c}$ > 7.5%), the addition of rosiglitazone, 2 or 4mg twice daily, significantly reduced HbA$_{1c}$ (-7 and -13%, respectively) and total daily insulin requirements (-7 and -12%, respectively) over 26 weeks.[48]

Pioglitazone

The published literature on pioglitazone remains less than for the other agents and much of the data is still in abstract form. However, recent papers have added important information since this class of drugs was last reviewed. Although a less potent agonist at the PPAR receptor, pioglitazone is comparable to rosiglitazone in improving glycaemic control, with significant reductions in FPG and HbA$_{1c}$ when used alone or in combination therapy.[15,42–44,49,86–89] One 26-week multicentre trial assessed the therapeutic effects of four doses of pioglitazone (7.5, 15, 30 or 45mg) administered as monotherapy versus placebo.[15] Significant dose-related reductions from baseline and compared with the placebo group were seen in FPG (-7 to -20% from baseline) and HbA$_{1c}$ (-3 to -9% from baseline) in all pioglitazone-treated groups. The magnitude of this response was greatest for those patients who were naïve to antidiabetic drug therapy and occurred relatively rapidly following commencement of the study medication – by week 2 for FPG and by week 14 for HbA$_{1c}$. Other trials with pioglitazone giving 30–45mg daily doses confirm this dose-related reduction in FBG and HbA$_{1c}$ by up to 25 and 12%, respectively, after 16 weeks of placebo-controlled therapy.[89] Table 6.2 compares two similarly designed 26-week trials of rosiglitazone and pioglitazone monotherapy. It should be noted, however, that in a non-randomized clinical setting, pioglitazone given at 45mg daily caused significantly more weight gain than rosiglitazone given at 8mg daily during 2–4 months of therapy.[86]

Combination therapy with pioglitazone, in addition to a sulphonylurea, metformin or insulin, benefits glycaemic control more than any of these agents used alone.[42–44,49] Pioglitazone, at 30mg daily, added to either metformin or sulphonylurea therapy in patients with poorly controlled diabetes (HbA$_{1c}$ $\geqslant$ 8%) significantly improved glycaemic control (HbA$_{1c}$ -12 and -6% from baseline, respectively).[42,43] Another 16-week trial com-

Table 6.2 Effects of rosiglitazone and pioglitazone – comparison of two randomized placebo-controlled trials over 26 weeks.

	HbA$_{1c}$* (%)	Total cholesterol[†]	LDL cholesterol[†]	HDL cholesterol[†]	Triglycerides[†]	Weight (change in kg)
Rosiglitazone (4mg bid)[‡]	−1.11	+13.5	+14.3	+13.9	+5.2	+3.3
Pioglitazone (30mg daily)[§]	−0.6	+3.3	+5.2	+12.2	−9.6	+1.29

*Change from baseline in drug-naïve patients.
[†]Percentage change from baselines.
[‡]From Phillips et al.[37]
[§]From Aronhoff et al.[15]

pared the addition of pioglitazone, 15 or 30mg daily, to a sulphonylurea (n = 560), metformin (n = 328) or insulin (n = 566). Combination therapy resulted in at least a 100% increase in the percentage of responders to treatment based upon predefined reductions in FBG and HbA$_{1c}$.[44]

Non-hypoglycaemic effects of the thiazolidinediones

In addition to elevated plasma glucose, Type 2 diabetes is associated with a cluster of other metabolic abnormalities, including obesity, dyslipidaemia, hypertension, and defects in clotting and fibrinolysis. These metabolic defects are strongly correlated with insulin resistance both in Type 2 diabetes and in pre-diabetes, and it is reasonable to propose that, along with improving glycaemic control, an insulin-sensitizer agent might have additional favourable effects on these parameters. These so-called non-hypoglycaemic effects of the thiazolidinediones have recently been reviewed by Parulkar et al.[90] Additional long-term clinical trials will still be needed to determine whether any demonstrated reduction in risk factors actually leads to less cardiovascular disease in patients with Type 2 diabetes.

Body weight

An important effect of the thiazolidinediones is the consistent dose-related increases in body weight seen across all members of the class.[15,43,44,49,86,89,91] Weight gain is seen when the thiazolidinediones are used as monotherapy, in combination with other oral agents (particularly sulphonylureas) or with insulin. The greater weight gain occurs with pioglitazone (up to 5% increase from baseline has been reported)[15,43,44,86,89] compared with rosiglitazone.[37,80,81,86] Although weight gain is correlated with the dose of pioglitazone, it is in fact more strongly associated with the inverse of any change in HbA_{1c}.[91] Despite the fact that weight gain is usually associated with increasing insulin resistance, thiazolidinediones clearly improve insulin sensitivity. Accurate measurement of insulin sensitivity by the glucose clamp method has not been published for any treatment period beyond 6 months.[13] This question can only be properly resolved by the appropriate clamp studies together with accurate measurements of regional fat distribution before and after much longer treatment periods. Current thinking is that weight gain may reflect the development of larger, more differentiated adipocytes (a known effect of the thiazolidinediones) with a shift in body fat distribution from central to less dysmetabolic subcutaneous stores. In addition, a proportion of weight gained may be secondary to fluid retention, as evidenced clinically by oedema in 5-8% of patients.[44,49,91] The clinical significance of treatment associated weight gain thus remains undetermined.

Lipid metabolism

Type 2 diabetes and the insulin-resistance syndrome are associated with a characteristic pattern of atherogenic dyslipidaemia, including an elevated plasma triglyceride level, low plasma high-density lipoprotein (HDL) levels and compositional changes in low-density lipoprotein (LDL) particles.[91–93] These compositional changes in LDL cholesterol result in a molecule which is smaller, denser and more triglyceride rich, and hence more susceptible to lipid oxidation. All the thiazolidinediones have been shown to increase HDL (12.2 and 11.8% with 30mg pioglitazone and 8mg rosiglitazone, respectively) and LDL, and hence total cholesterol levels.[37,51–54,80,95] However, this increase is predominantly in the larger, more buoyant particles of LDL, which may be less atherogenic than the smaller, denser particles.

While pioglitazone appears to have a beneficial effect on plasma triglycerides (30mg of pioglitazone reduces triglycerides by a mean of 9.6% over 26 weeks), rosiglitazone has been shown to be either neutral or to cause some elevation in both triglycerides and LDL cholesterol.[37,80,86,89] As clinical experience grows, the choice of which insulin sensitizer to prescribe may depend less on their glycaemic benefit and potential side effects (both of which are approximately equal between the two drugs), and more on balancing the effects on body weight and lipid profiles in the individual patient.

Blood pressure and vascular reactivity

In animal studies, both pioglitazone and rosiglitazone have been shown to reduce blood pressure and improve vascular reactivity and endothelial function.[55–57] As yet, there are no human data available for pioglitazone.

Rosiglitazone, given at 4mg twice daily, significantly reduced diastolic blood pressure (−2.7mmHg, p = 0.0046) compared with glibenclamide in patients treated for 1 year.[58]

Urinary albumin excretion

Microalbuminuria is a marker of impaired vascular integrity, early nephropathy and a predictor of cardiovascular disease. Pioglitazone and rosiglitazone significantly reduce urinary albumin excretion in patients with Type 2 diabetes.[59,60] Whether these drugs will have a role in delaying the progression of diabetic nephropathy, perhaps as useful adjuncts to angiotensin-converting enzyme (ACE) inhibitors, remains to be determined.

Safety

Minor side effects noted for the thiazolidinediones include a slight reduction in plasma haemoglobin, haematocrit, platelets and neutrophils, and the development of peripheral oedema, but these have not yet proved to be clinically significant. During the clinical development of troglitazone, reversible elevations in serum ALT (greater than three times the upper limit of normal) occurred in 2% of troglitazone-treated patients compared with 0.6% of placebo-treated patients. Following initial licensing in the USA and Japan, a number of cases of idiosyncratic hepatotoxicity, associated with death or transplant requirement in c. 1 in 60,000 patients treated, have been reported.[96-98] Troglitazone was voluntarily withdrawn from the UK market in 1997 and the Food and Drug Administration (FDA) recommended its withdrawal from the US market in March 2000.[33] Whether or not hepatotoxicity is a class effect remains to be fully established. Pooled data from more than 4500 patients treated with rosiglitazone showed a similar proportion of patients with ALT greater than three times the upper limit of normal in placebo/active comparator-treated and rosiglitazone-treated groups.[99] However, since marketing, two possible rosiglitazone-related cases of hepatotoxicity have been reported.[100,101] Both cases involved patients with co-morbid conditions and concomitant use of other medications, and the causative role of rosiglitazone remains undetermined. In fact, a patient who developed troglitazone-related hepatitis was subsequently treated with rosiglitazone without difficulty.[102] To date, there are no reports of significant hepatotoxicity in pioglitazone-treated patients. In pooled data from more than 4500 patients treated with pioglitazone the frequency of adverse events was similar to those of the placebo groups.[91] Current recommendations are that liver enzymes should be checked prior to the initiation of therapy, every 2 months for the first 12 months of treatment and periodically thereafter. Thiazolidinediones should not be used in patients with evidence of liver disease at baseline.

Cardiac hypertrophy has been noted in rodents given high doses of thiazolidinediones.[103] Assessment (by echocardiogram) of 104 patients treated with rosiglitazone, 4mg twice daily for 52 weeks, did not demonstrate any adverse changes in cardiac structure or function.[104] Similarly, pioglitazone does not adversely effect cardiac mass or function.[91] The thiazolidinediones are, however, currently contraindicated in patients with advanced heart failure because of their tendency to increase plasma volume.

Rosiglitazone has been shown to be effective in terms of glycaemic control, and safe in elderly patients (over 65 years) and in patients with mild to moderate renal failure (creatinine clearance 30-80ml/min), with no dose adjustment required.[105,106]

Drug interactions

No significant drug interactions have been reported to date for either rosiglitazone or pioglitazone. Rosiglitazone does not interfere with the cytochrome P_{450} system and has been shown not to interact with ranitidine, nifedipine, digoxin or the oral contraceptive pill.[107,108] Similarly, pioglitazone does not induce or inhibit hepatic enzymes and has been shown not to interact with warfarin, glipizide, glibenclamide, metformin, digoxin, prednisolone or oestrogen/progesterone combinations as used in the oral contraceptive pill and hormone replacement therapy.[109,110]

The thiazolidinediones have not been formally studied in paediatric, pregnant or breast-feeding populations and should not be administered to these groups.

Clinical use of the glitazones

While the current licensing restrictions must be observed, it is clear that the glitazones cannot play a significant role in diabetes care until these limitations are modified (Table 6.3). Based on the clinical research programmes for the glitazones, and based on post-marketing clinical experience both in the US and elsewhere, there is a clear rationale for the use of these agents early in the course of Type 2 diabetes. Monotherapy is therefore a likely future indication. Previous research experience has shown that there is a c. 20-25% non-response rate to the glitazones (in terms of plasma glucose). It is not completely clear which patients do not respond, but it is likely that those patients in whom insulin resistance rather than loss of insulin secretion is the major defect will benefit more from treatment. It would be helpful in future clinical care to be able to

Table 6.3 Thiazolidinediones – potential spectrum for use.

- Type 2 diabetes mellitus
  Monotherapy
  Combination with sulphonylureas
  Combination with metformin
  Triple combination oral therapy
  Combination with insulin
- Pre-diabetes (impaired glucose tolerance, impaired fasting glycaemia)
- As cardiovascular protection in the insulin resistance syndrome
- Other conditions associated with insulin resistance (e.g. polycystic ovarian syndrome)

conveniently measure both insulin resistance and insulin secretion with a view to early, directed selection of first-line monotherapy, after diet and exercise have been addressed. To that end the present authors, and others, have proposed mathematical models based on the glucose and insulin responses during the oral glucose tolerance test (OGTT) that allow insulin sensitivity and secretion to be estimated.[111–113] Beyond monotherapy, there is clear evidence for combination therapy, with either sulphonylureas or metformin, which is currently permitted. There is a strong case however for the earlier combination with metformin or with sulphonylurea, without a restriction to those with intolerance to either. Taking all the clinical evidence into account, the most logical first-line combination would be with metformin. Triple combination should be studied prospectively and is also logical on the basis of complementary mechanisms of action. Insulin combination therapy has been studied in detail and is a completely logical therapeutic step in patients with more advanced Type 2 diabetes. Although there has been some concern about increased fluid retention in some of these patients, the published evidence from this across the class of glitazones is small and would appear to be greatly outweighed by a range of positive effects, particularly on glycaemic control and insulin dose.

Most controversial is the question of use of the glitazones in pre-diabetic or non-diabetic subjects with insulin resistance. Two possible benefits underlie such a strategy: (1) the prevention of diabetes itself; (2) the prevention of atherosclerotic cardiovascular disease. Diabetes prevention is now being seriously considered and is under study by the National Institute of Health (NIH) (The Diabetes Prevention Program), and will be the subject of several future drug trials.[114] Unfortunately, the NIH study included an arm with troglitazone that later had to be discontinued when the potential for hepatotoxicity was discovered. In fact, the hypothesis that reduction of insulin resistance in pre-diabetic subjects could prevent diabetes had not formally been tested until recently. The recently reported Finnish Diabetes Prevention Study has clearly shown the bene-

fits of a committed outpatient diet and exercise regime in preventing progression from impaired glucose tolerance (IGT) to diabetes in a group of
523 subjects over a mean follow-up period of 3.2 years.[115] Troglitazone
has been shown to improve insulin resistance and glucose tolerance in
IGT[16] and in the polycystic ovary syndrome.[116] It is very likely that the
other glitazones, including those in development, will have similar beneficial effects in these pre-diabetic conditions, particularly if combined with
a diet and exercise strategy along the lines of the Finnish study. This is
another important potential future indication for the glitazones.

The prevention of atherosclerotic cardiovascular disease is a further
extension of the concept of diabetes prevention. Much evidence now
links insulin resistance with atherosclerosis, although a single clear
prospective trial of this hypothesis is lacking. Several epidemiological
studies, most recently the DECODE study, have shown that the increased
cardiovascular risk begins very early in the evolution of hyperglycaemia
in diabetes.[117] Thus, the cardiovascular risk rises steeply once the 2 hour
glucose (in the OGTT) rises above the IGT threshold. The results of the
DECODE study (and other similar but smaller studies) support early intervention to improve glycaemia in IGT and diabetes on the basis of cardiovascular risk.[114] A number of trials are now in progress to test the
potential for the glitazones to prevent cardiovascular disease in high-risk
subjects with diabetes. It is conceivable, but would have to be tested in
trials, that insulin-sensitizer drugs might be used in patients with cardiovascular disease alone, or features of the metabolic syndrome alone,
without abnormal fasting or post-challenge glucose concentrations. While
the upfront costs to the National Health Service (NHS) of the thiazolidinediones are substantially greater than those of either the sulphonylureas or
metformin (Table 6.4), these costs may potentially be outweighed by

Table 6.4 Comparison of costs of oral hypoglycaemic agents (based on a
30-day month).

Oral hypoglycaemic agent	Cost per month (£)	Cost per annum (£)
Metformin (2g daily)	3.25	38.90
Gliclazide (160mg twice daily)	12.50	150.00
Pioglitazone (30mg daily)	42.80	513.80
Rosiglitazone (8mg daily)	58.50	702.00

NICE suggests that, based on similar glucose-lowering effectiveness, the thiazolidinediones may be a
less cost-effective option than sulphonylureas or metformin, although issues of tolerability and other non-
glycaemic benefits of the glitazones may be taken into account when prescribing.

long-term cardiovascular benefits. In summary, it is likely that the indications for eventual use of the glitazones will be expanded far beyond current regulatory limitations. Monotherapy, free combination therapy, triple combination and combination with insulin are all realistic prospects. The potential exists for use in pre-diabetic subjects with the metabolic syndrome, both for the prevention of diabetes itself and its cardiovascular complications. These latter indications will need to be underpinned with clear evidence from prospective clinical trials.

References

1. Polonsky KS, Sturis J, Bell GI. Non-insulin dependent diabetes mellitus – a genetically programmed failure of the beta cell to compensate for insulin resistance. New Engl J Med 1996; 334:777–83.

2. Nolan JJ, Olefsky JM. Insulin action and insulin resistance in NIDDM. In: Draznin B, Rizza R, editors. Clinical research in diabetes and obesity: volume II: diabetes and obesity. The Humana Press: NJ, USA, 1997:137–58.

3. DeFronzo RA, Bonadonna RC, Ferrannini E. Pathogenesis of NIDDM: a balanced overview. Diabetologia 1992; 35:389–97.

4. Reaven GM. Role of insulin resistance in human disease. Diabetes 1988; 37:1595–607.

5. DeFronzo RA. Pharmacologic therapy for Type 2 diabetes mellitus. Ann Intern Med 1999; 131: 281–303.

6. Fujita T, Sugiyama Y, Taketomi S, et al. Reduction of insulin resistance in obese and/or diabetic animals by 3[-4-(1-methylcyclohexylmethoxy)benzyl]-thiazolidine-2,4-dione (ADD-3870, U63287, ciglitazone), a new antidiabetic agent. Diabetes 1983; 32:804–10.

7. Fujiwara T, Yoshioka S, Yoshioka T, et al. Characterisation of a new antidiabetic agent, CS-045: studies in KK and ob/ob mice and

Zucker fatty rats. Diabetes 1988; 37:1549–88.

8. Ikeda H, Taketomi S, Sugiyama Y, et al. Effects of pioglitazone on glucose and lipid metabolism in normal and insulin resistant animals. Arz-Forsch/Drug Res 1990; 40:156–62.

9. Oakes ND, Kennedy CJ, Jenkins AB, et al. A new antidiabetic agent, BRL 49653, reduces lipid availability and improves insulin action and glucoregulation in the rat. Diabetes 1994; 43:1203–10.

10. Day C. Thiazolidinediones: a new class of antidiabetic drugs. Diabet Med 1999; 16:179–92.

11. Murphy E, Nolan JJ. Insulin sensitiser drugs. Expl Opin Invest Drugs 2000; 9:1346–61.

12. Olefsky JM. Treatment of insulin resistance with peroxisome proliferator-activated receptor γ agonists. J Clin Invest 2000; 106: 467–72.

13. Maggs DG, Buchanan TA, Burant CF, et al. Metabolic effects of troglitazone monotherapy in Type 2 diabetes mellitus. A randomized, double-blind, placebo-controlled trial. Ann Intern Med 1998; 128:176–85.

14. Patel J, Anderson RJ, Rappaport EB. Rosiglitazone monotherapy improves glycaemic control inpatients with Type 2 diabetes: a twelve-week, randomized, placebo-

controlled study. Diabetes Obes Metab 1999; 1:165–72.

15. Aronoff S, Rosenblatt S, Braithwaite S, et al. Pioglitazone hydrochloride monotherapy improves glycaemic control in the treatment of patients with type 2 diabetes: a 6–month randomized placebo-controlled dose-response study. The Pioglitazone 001 Study Group. Diabetes Care 2000; 23:1605–11.

16. Nolan JJ, Ludvik B, Beerdsen P, et al. Improvement in glucose tolerance and insulin resistance in obese subjects treated with troglitazone. New Engl J Med 1994; 331:1188–93.

17. Antonucci T, Whitcomb R, McLain R, Lockwood D. Impaired glucose tolerance is normalized by treatment with the thiazolidinedione troglitazone. Diabetes Care 1997; 20:188–93.

18. Berkowitz K, Peters R, Kjos S, et al. Effect of troglitazone on insulin sensitivity and pancreatic beta-cell function in women at high risk for NIDDM. Diabetes 1996; 45: 1572–9.

19. Dunaif A, Scott D, Finegood D, et al. The insulin-sensitizing agent troglitazone improves metabolic and reproductive abnormalities in the polycystic ovary syndrome. J Clin Endocr Metab 1996; 81: 3299–306.

20. Ehtisham S, Barrett TG, Shaw NJ. Type 2 diabetes mellitus in UK children – an emerging problem. Diabet Med 2000; 17:867–71.

21. Fagot-Campagna A, Naravan KM, Imperatore G. Type 2 diabetes in children. Br Med J 2001; 322:377–8.

22. Stratton IM, Adler AI, Neil HA. Association of glycaemia with macrovascular and microvascular complications of type 2 diabetes (UKPDS 35): prospective observational study. Br Med J 2000; 321:405–12.

23. Turner RC, Cull CA, Frighi V, Holman RR. Glycemic control with diet, sulfonylurea, metformin, or insulin in patients with Type 2 diabetes mellitus: progressive requirement for multiple therapies (UKPDS 49). UK Prospective Diabetes Study (UKPDS) Group. J Am Med Ass 1999; 281:2005–12.

24. Matthaei S, Stumvoll M, Kellerer M, Häring HA. Pathophysiology and pharmacological treatment of insulin resistance. Endocr Rev 2000; 21:585–618.

25. Campbell IW. Antidiabetic drugs present and future: will improving insulin resistance benefit cardiovascular risk in Type 2 diabetes mellitus? Drugs 2000; 60: 1018–29.

26. Effect of intensive blood-glucose control with metformin on complications in overweight patients with Type 2 diabetes (UKPDS 34). UK Prospective Diabetes Study (UKPDS) Group. Lancet 1998; 352:854–65.

27. Turner RC. The UK Prospective Diabetes Study. A review. Diabetes Care 1998; 21:C35–C38.

28. Pyorala K, Pedersen TR, Kjekshus J, et al. Cholesterol lowering with simvastatin improves prognosis of diabetic patients with coronary heart disease. Diabetes Care 1997; 20:614–21.

29. Goldberg RB, Mellies MJ, Sacks FM, et al. Cardiovascular events and their reduction with pravastatin in diabetic and glucose-intolerant myocardial infarction survivors with average cholesterol levels: subgroup analyses in the cholesterol and recurrent events (CARE) trial. Circulation 1998; 98:2513–19.

30. Long-term Intervention with Pravastatin in Ischaemic disease (LIPID) Study Group. Prevention of cardiovascular events and death with pravastatin in patients

with coronary heart disease and a broad range of initial cholesterol levels. New Engl J Med 1998; 339:1349–57.

31. Effect of fenofibrate on progression of coronary-artery disease in Type 2 diabetes: the Diabetes Atherosclerosis Intervention Study, a randomised study. Lancet 2001; 357:905–10.

32. Heart Outcomes Prevention Evaluation Study Investigators. Effects of ramipril on cardiovascular and microvascular outcomes in people with diabetes mellitus: results of the HOPE study and MICRO-HOPE substudy. Lancet 2000; 355:253–9.

33. US Department of Health and Human Services. Rezulin to be withdrawn from the market. March 21, 2000.

34. National Institute for Clinical Excellence. Guidance on the use of rosiglitazone for Type 2 diabetes mellitus. www.nice.org.uk.

35. National Institute for Clinical Excellence. Guidance on the use of pioglitazone for Type 2 diabetes mellitus. www.nice.org.uk.

36. Grunberger G, Dole JF, Freed MI. Rosiglitazone monotherapy significantly lowers HbA1c levels in treatment-naïve Type 2 diabetic patients. Diabetes 2000; 49:A109, 441.

37. Phillips LS, Grunberger G, Miller E, et al. Once- and twice-daily dosing with rosiglitazone improves glycaemic control in patients with Type 2 diabetes. Diabetes Care 2001; 24:308–15.

38. Wolffenbuttel BHR, Gomis R, Squatrito S, et al. Addition of low-dose rosiglitazone to sulphonylurea therapy improves glycaemic control in Type 2 diabetic patients. Diabet Med 2000; 17:40–7.

39. Fonseca V, Rosenstock J, Pat-wardhan R, Salzman A. Effect of metformin and rosiglitazone combination therapy in patients with Type 2 diabetes mellitus. J Am Med Ass 2000; 283:1695–702.

40. Jones T, Jones NP, Sautter M. Addition of rosiglitazone to metformin is effective in obese, insulin-resistant patients with Type 2 diabetes. Diabetologia 2000; 43:A191, 735.

41. Jones NP, Mather R, Owen S, et al. Long-term efficacy of rosiglitazone as monotherapy or in combination with metformin. Diabetologia 2000; 43:A192, 736.

42. Schneider R, Egan J, Houser V. Combination therapy with pioglitazone and sulphonylurea in patients with Type 2 diabetes. Diabetes 1999; 48:A106, 0458.

43. Einhorn D, Rendell M, Rosenzweig J, et al. Pioglitazone hydrochloride in combination with metformin in the treatment of Type 2 diabetes mellitus: a randomized, placebo-controlled study. The Pioglitazone 027 Study Group. Clin Ther 2000; 22: 1395–409.

44. Lebrezzi R, Egan JW, Study Group Pioglitazone 010, 014 & 027. The HbA1c and blood glucose response to pioglitazone in combination with another antidiabetic agent in patients with Type 2 diabetes. Diabetes 2000; 49: A114, 463.

45. Schwartz S, Raskin P, Fonseca V, Graveline JF, for the Troglitazone and Exogenous Insulin Study Group. Effect of troglitazone in insulin-treated patients with Type 2 diabetes. New Engl J Med 1998; 338:861–6.

46. Buse JB, Gumbiner B, Mathias NP, et al. Troglitazone use in insulin-treated Type 2 diabetic patients. The Troglitazone Insulin Study Group. Diabetes Care 1998; 21:1455–61.

47. Leiter L, Ross S, Halle JP, Tomovici A. Efficacy and safety of troglitazone in Type 2 diabetic patients inadequately controlled on insulin therapy. Diabetes 1999; 48:A115, 0495.

48. Raskin P, Dole JF, Rappaport E. Rosiglitazone improves glycaemic control in poorly controlled insulin treated Type 2 diabetes. Diabetes 1999; 48:A94, 0404.

49. Rubin C, Egan J, Schneider R. Combination therapy with pioglitazone and insulin in patients with type 2 diabetes. Diabetes 1999; 48:A110, 0474.

50. Inzucchi SE, Maggs DG, Spollett GR, et al. Efficacy and metabolic effects of metformin and troglitazone in Type 2 diabetes mellitus. New Engl J Med 1998; 338: 867–72.

51. Tack CJJ, Smits P, Demacker PNM, Stalenhoef AFH. Troglitazone decreases the proportion of small, dense LDL and increases the resistance of LDL to oxidation in obese subjects. Diabetes Care 1998; 21:796–9.

52. Brockley MR, Egan JW, Zhu E. The effect of pioglitazone on the lipid profile based on the baseline triglyceride and HDL levels. Diabetes 2000; 49:A354, 1484.

53. Zhu E, Egan JW. The effect of lipid reducing drugs on the serum lipid profile in pioglitazone-treated patients. Diabetes 2000; 49:A366, 1539.

54. Shaffer S, Rubin CJ, Zhu E, Study Group Pioglitazone. The effect of pioglitazone on the lipid profile in patients with Type 2 diabetes. Diabetes 2000; 49:A125, 508.

55. Walker AB, Naderali EK, Chattington PD, et al. Differential vasoactive effects of the insulin sensitizers rosiglitazone (BRL 49653) and troglitazone on human small arteries in vitro. Diabetes 1998; 47:810–14.

56. Walker AB, Chattington PD, Buckingham RE, Williams G. The thiazolidinedione rosiglitazone (BRL-49653) lowers blood pressure and protects against impairment of endothelial function in Zucker fatty rats. Diabetes 1999; 47:1448–53.

57. Kotchen TA, Zhang HY, Reddy S, Hoffmann RG. Effect of pioglitazone on vascular reactivity in vivo and in vitro. Am J Physiol 1996; 270:R660–R666.

58. Bakris GL, Dole JF, Porter LE, et al. Rosiglitazone improves blood pressure in patients with Type 2 diabetes mellitus. Diabetes 2000; 49:A96, 388.

59. Nakamura T, Ushiyama C, Shimada N, et al. Comparative effects of pioglitazone, glibenclamide, and voglibose on urinary endothelin-1 and albumin excretion in diabetes patients. J Diabetes Complic 2000; 14: 250–4.

60. Lebowitz HE, Dole FJ, Patwardhan R, et al. Rosiglitazone monotherapy is effective in patients with type 2 diabetes. J Clin Endocr Metab 2001; 86: 280–8.

61. Lemberger T, Desvergne B, Wahli W. Peroxisome proliferator activated receptors: a nuclear receptor signalling pathway in lipid physiology. Ann Rev Cell Devl Biol 1996; 12:353–63.

62. Schoonjans K, Peinado-Onsurbe J, Lefebvre AM, et al. PPARalpha and PPARgamma activators direct a distinct tissue-specific transcriptional response via a PPRE in the lipoprotein lipase gene. Eur Molec Biol Org J 1996; 15:5336–48.

63. Tontonoz P, Graves RA, Budavari AI, et al. Adipocyte-specific transcription factor ARF6 is a heterodimeric complex of two nuclear hormone receptors, PPAR

gamma and RXR alpha. Nucleic Acids Res 1994; 22:5628–34.

64. Castelein H, Gulick T, Declercq PE, et al. The peroxisome proliferator activated receptor regulates malic enzyme gene expression. J Biol Chem 1994; 269:26,754–8.

65. Keller H, Dreyer C, Medin J, et al. Fatty acids and retinoids control lipid metabolism through activation of peroxisome proliferator-activated receptor-retinoid X receptor heterodimers. Proc Natl Acad Sci USA 1993; 90:2160–4.

66. Lehmann JM, Moore LB, Smith-Oliver TA, et al. An antidiabetic thiazolidinedione is a high affinity ligand for peroxisome proliferator-activated receptor γ (PPARγ). J Biol Chem 1995; 270:12,953–6.

67. Nolte RT, Wisely GB, Westin S, et al. Ligand binding and co-activator assembly of the peroxisome proliferator-activated receptor gamma. Nature 1998; 395: 137–43.

68. Gelman L, Zhou G, Fajas L, et al. p300 interacts with the N- and C-terminal part of PPARgamma2 in a ligand-independent and -dependent manner, respectively. J Biol Chem 1999; 274:7681–8.

69. Zhu Y, Qi C, Calandra C, et al. Cloning and identification of mouse steroid receptor coactivator-1 (mSRC-1), as a coactivator of peroxisome proliferator-activated receptor γ. Gene Expr 1996; 6:185–95.

70. Zhu Y, Kan L, Qi C, et al. Isolation and characterization of peroxisome proliferator-activated receptor (PPAR) interacting protein (PRIP) a coactivator for PPAR. J Biol Chem 2000; 275:13,510–16.

71. Zhu Y, Qi C, Jain M, et al. Isolation and characterization of PBP, a protein that interacts with peroxisome proliferator-activated receptor. J Biol Chem 1997; 272:25,500–6.

72. Braissant O, Foufelle F, Scotto C, et al. Differential expression of peroxisome proliferator-activated receptors (PPARS): tissue distribution of PPAR-alpha, -beta, -gamma in the adult rat. Endocrinology 1996; 137:354–66.

73. Roden M, Price TB, Perseghin G, et al. Mechanism of free fatty acid-induced insulin resistance in humans. J Clin Invest 1996; 97: 2859–65.

74. Bergman RN, Ader M. Free fatty acids and pathogenesis of Type 2 diabetes mellitus. Trends Endocr Metab 2000; 11:351–6.

75. Yamasaki Y, Kawamori R, Wasada T, et al. Pioglitazone (AD-4833) ameliorates insulin resistance in patients with NIDDM. AD-4833 Glucose Clamp Study Group, Japan. Tohoku J Expl Med 1997; 183:173–83.

76. Chao L, Marcus-Samuels B, Mason MM, et al. Adipose tissue is required for the antidiabetic, but not for the hypolipidemic, effect of thiazolidiediones. J Clin Invest 2000; 106:1221–8.

77. Kahn CR, Chen L, Cohen SE. Unraveling the mechanism of action of thiazolidinediones. J Clin Invest 2000; 106:1305–7.

78. Steppan CM, Bailey ST, Bhat S, et al. The hormone resistin links obesity to diabetes. Nature 2001; 409:307–12.

79. Flier JS. The missing link with obesity. Nature 2001; 409:292–3.

80. Raskin P, Rappaport EB, Cole ST, et al. Rosiglitazone short-term monotherapy lowers fasting and post-prandial glucose in patients with Type 2 diabetes. Diabetologia 2000; 43:278–84.

81. Nolan JJ, Jones JP, Patwardhan R, Deacon LF. Rosiglitazone taken once daily is effective in the treatment of Type 2 diabetes mellitus. Diabet Med 2000; 17: 287–94.

82. Greene DA, Viberti GF, Berry RA, et al. A diabetes outcome progression trial (ADOPT) of long-term rosiglitazone, metformin and glyburide monotherapy in drug-naïve patients. Diabetes 2000; 49:A343, 1435.

83. Mori Y, Murakawa Y, Okada K, et al. Effect of troglitazone on body fat distribution in type 2 diabetic subjects. Diabetes Care 1999; 6:908–12.

84. Kawai T, Takei I, Oguma Y, et al. Effects of troglitazone on fat distribution in the treatment of male Type 2 diabetes. Metabolism 1999; 48:1102–7.

85. Charbonnel B, Lonnqvist F, Jones NP, et al. Rosiglitazone is superior to glyburide in reducing fasting plasma glucose after 1 year of treatment in Type 2 diabetic patients. Diabetes 1999; 48:A114, 494.

86. King AB. A comparison in a clinical setting of the efficacy and side effects of three thiazolidinediones. Diabetes Care 2000; 23:557.

87. Göke B. Pioglitazone is superior to acarbose in improving glycaemic control and dyslipidaemia in patients with Type 2 diabetes. Diabetologia 2000; 43:A193, 740.

88. Yu S. Effect of pioglitazone on blood glucose following an oral glucose challenge. Diabetes 2000; 49:A352, 1476.

89. Mathisen A, Geerlof J, Houser V. The effect of pioglitazone on glucose control and lipid profile in patients with Type 2 diabetes. Diabetes 1999; 48:441.

90. Parulkar AA, Pendergrass ML, Granda-Ayala R, et al, Nonhypoglycemic effects of thiazolidinediones. Ann Intern Med 2001; 134:61–71.

91. Aronoff SL. Adverse events with pioglitazone HCL. Diabetes 2000; 49:A340, 1425.

92. Yki-Jarvinen H. Management of Type 2 diabetes mellitus and cardiovascular risk: lessons from intervention trials. Drugs 2000; 60:975–83.

93. Howard BV. Insulin resistance and lipid metabolism. Am J Cardiol 1999; 84:28J-32J.

94. Reaven GM, Chen Y-DI, Jeppesen J, et al. Insulin resistance and hyperinsulinaemia in individuals with small, dense low density lipoprotein particles. J Clin Invest 1993; 92:141–6.

95. Fonseca VA, Valiquett TR, Huang SM, et al. Troglitazone monotherapy improves glycemic control in patients with Type 2 diabetes mellitus: a randomized, controlled study. J Clin Endocr Metab 1998; 83:3169–75.

96. Gitlin N, Neil J, Spurr CL, et al. Two cases of severe clinical and histologic hepatotoxicity associated with troglitazone. Ann Intern Med 1998; 129:36–8.

97. Neuschwander-Tetri BA, Isley WL, Oki JC, et al. Troglitazone-induced hepatic failure leading to liver transplantation. Ann Intern Med 1998; 129:38–41.

98. Watkins PB, Whitcomb RW. Hepatic dysfunction associated with troglitazone. New Engl J Med 1998; 338:916–17.

99. Salzman A. Rosiglitazone is not associated with hepatotoxicity. Diabetologia 1999; 42:A3, 8.

100. Al-Salman J, Arjomand H, Kemp DG, Mittal M. Hepatocellular injury in a patient receiving rosiglitazone. Ann Intern Med 2000; 132:121–4.

101. Forman LM, Simmons DA, Diamond RH. Hepatic failure in a patient taking rosiglitazone. Ann Intern Med 2000; 132:118–21.

102. Lenhard MJ, Funk WB. Failure to develop hepatic injury from rosiglitazone in a patient with a

history of troglitazone-induced hepatitis. Diabetes Care 2001; 24:168–9.

103. Williams GD, Deldar A, Jordan WH, et al. Subchronic toxicity of the thiazolidinedione Tanabe-174 (LY282449) in the rat and the dog. Diabetes 1993; 42:186A.

104. St John Sutton M, Dole JF, Rappaport EB. Rosiglitazone does not adversely affect cardiac structure or function in patients with Type 2 diabetes. Diabetes 1999; 48: A102, 0438.

105. Beebe K, Patel J. Rosiglitazone is effective and well tolerated in patients ⩾ 65 years with Type 2 diabetes. Diabetes 1999; 48: A111, 0479.

106. Agrawal A, Jones NP, Sautter M. Rosiglitazone added to a sulphonlyurea in patients with Type 2 diabetes and mild-to-moderate renal impairment. Diabetologia 2000; 43:A191, 734.

107. Thompson KA, Miller AK, Inglis AML, et al. Rosiglitazone does not markedly alter CYP3A4–mediated drug metabolism. Diabetologia 1999; 42:A227, 852.

108. Balfour JA, Plosker GL. Rosiglitazone. Drugs 1999; 57:921–30.

109. Gillies PS, Dunn CJ. Pioglitazone. Drugs 2000; 60:333–43.

110. Glazer NB, Cheatham WW. Thiazolidinediones for Type 2 diabetes. No evidence exists that pioglitazone induces hepatic cytochrome P450 isoform CYP3A4. Br Med J 2001; 322: 235–6.

111. Mari A, Pacini G, Murphy E, et al. A model-based method for assessing insulin sensitivity from the oral glucose tolerance test. Diabetes Care 2001; 24:539–48.

112. Matsuda M, DeFronzo RA. Insulin sensitivity indices obtained from oral glucose tolerance testing: comparison with the euglycaemic insulin clamp. Diabetes Care 1999; 22:1462–70.

113. Stumvoll M, Mitrakou A, Pimenta W, et al. Use of the oral glucose tolerance test to assess insulin release and insulin sensitivity. Diabetes Care 2000; 23:295–301.

114. The Diabetes Prevention Program Research Group. The Diabetes Prevention Program. Design and methods for a clinical trial in the prevention of Type 2 diabetes. Diabetes Care 1999; 22:623–34.

115. Tuomilehto J, Lindström J, Erikkson JG, et al. for The Finnish Diabetes Prevention Study Group. Prevention of Type 2 diabetes mellitus by changes in lifestyle among subjects with impaired glucose tolerance. New Engl J Med 2001; 344:1343–50.

116. Ehrmann DA, Schneider DJ, Sobel BE, et al. Troglitazone improves defects in insulin action, insulin secretion, ovarian steroidogenesis, and fibrinolysis in women with polycystic ovary syndrome. J Clin Endocr Metab 1997; 82:2108–16.

117. DECODE. Consequences of the new diagnostic criteria for diabetes in older men and women. DECODE Study (Diabetes Epidemiology: Collaborative Analysis of Diagnostic Criteria in Europe). Diabetes Care 1999; 22:1667–71.

118. Charles MA, Balkau B, Vauzelle-Kervroedan F, et al. Revision of diagnostic criteria for diabetes. Lancet 1996; 348:1657–8.

7

What is the role of designer insulins (insulin analogues) in clinical practice?

Simon R Heller

Introduction

The last 10 years has seen a change in the insulin market that may soon become a revolution. Although many different formulations were available before 1990, the basic insulin structure, whether animal or human, remained unaltered. The introduction of human insulin bought little clinical benefit but the genetic engineering techniques used in its manufacture afforded insulin manufacturers freedom to manipulate the insulin molecule in any way they chose. Two rapid-acting analogues are now widely available, and a fixed-dose mixture combining a rapid-acting analogue and isophane insulin is proving extremely popular. The first long-acting insulin preparation is already available in the USA and it, and others, will shortly be launched in Europe. Is their popularity justified by the evidence? What are the true clinical benefits of the analogue insulins and in what situations should they be used? Can insulin analogues be used with confidence about their safety? These are some of the questions that will be addressed in this chapter. It is not a systematic review but as many recent papers as possible have been searched for. Nevertheless, limitations of space demands selection in those cited and readers also need to take into account positive bias, since studies with negative results will tend to be published either later or not at all.

The need for insulin analogues

It is only recently that most clinicians have recognized the need for better methods of insulin delivery. For the first 50 years or so after the discovery of insulin, most people with diabetes took either one or two injections each day, often with a mixture of quick-acting soluble and medium-acting isophane or lente, and tried to keep the urine sugar free. However, the advent of home blood glucose monitoring and the evidence that tight metabolic control could prevent or delay diabetic microvascular complications[1,2] led to a push to use insulin more intensively to achieve tighter glucose targets. As patients and their doctors struggled with conventional insulin to achieve near normoglycaemia, so its limitations became increasingly apparent. Those who attempted this with twice-daily insulin often suffered major hypoglycaemic episodes. Even patients who were switched to basal bolus regimens were prone to hypoglycaemia, particularly if they strived for tight glycaemic control. Studies have showed that intermittent injections with conventional insulins produce insulin profiles that bear little resemblance to those of people without diabetes (Figure 7.1).[3,4] It seems that the only way that patients can safely achieve tight glycaemic control is to provide them with delivery systems that produce a more physiological insulin profile.

The challenge to the insulin manufacturers has been to solve two main problems. First, soluble insulin, when injected subcutaneously, is absorbed relatively slowly with a resulting slow rise and fall in concentration compared to the sharp insulin peak produced by pancreatic beta cell secretion in response to eating. This leads to high postprandial

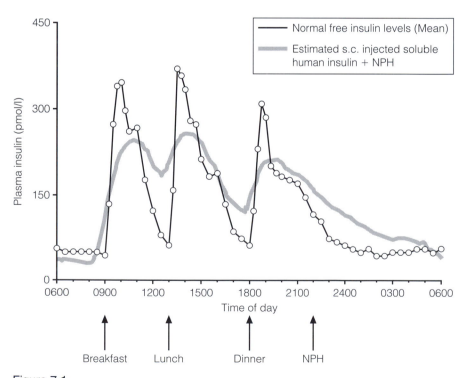

Figure 7.1

Insulin profiles in patients treated intensively with multiple subcutaneous injections of conventional insulin. Insulin profiles redrawn from Rizza et al.,[3] and Polonsky et al.[4]

glucose levels and a susceptibility to hypoglycaemia in the post-absorptive period, particularly just before the next meal. Second, between meals and at night the pancreatic beta cells release insulin at a constant, low rate to maintain a basal concentration with a flat profile. Unfortunately, none of the conventional isophane or lente preparations are absorbed from subcutaneous depots at a constant rate and so produce concentrations that peak some hours after injection. Furthermore, their absorption rates show considerable intra- and inter-individual variation. Both of these limitations lead to inappropriate, and often unpredictable, hyperinsulinaemia at night and a subsequent high risk of hypoglycaemia.

Quick-acting insulin analogues

The unphysiological insulin profiles exhibited by conventional insulin structure of any species is due to the tendency of insulin molecules to self-associate into hexamers at high concentrations (Figure 7.2).[5] This

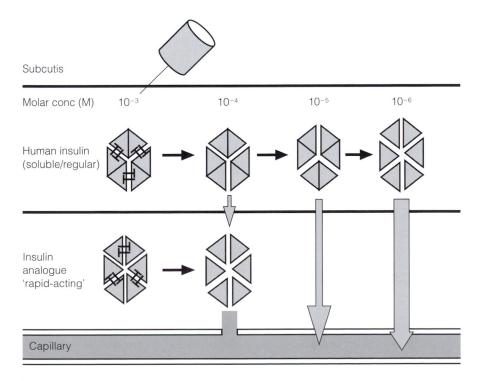

Figure 7.2

Representation of absorption of conventional soluble and rapid-acting insulin analogue after subcutaneous injection.

property is probably useful in packaging insulin into granules within the beta cell but becomes an important limitation when preparing a pharmaceutical preparation for therapeutic use. Thus, soluble insulin after subcutaneous (sc) injection remains at the injection site for minutes to hours rather than being absorbed rapidly into the bloodstream. The development of genetic engineering using rDNA technology allowed insulin chemists to manipulate the insulin molecule and alter its physiochemical characteristics.[6] One of the first insulin analogues with less self-aggregation, insulin B10^{Asp}, was produced by Novo Nordisk in the 1980s.[7] Although this showed promise in early trials it was withdrawn after studies demonstrated increased rates of mammary tumours in rats.[8] This event highlighted the important fact that altering the structure of the insulin molecule is not without potential risk (the issue of safety is considered later).

Eli Lilly & Co became interested in the structural homology of insulin-like growth factor (IGF)-1 for other reasons since, in contrast to insulin, IGF-1 has no tendency to self-aggregation. This is related to a different amino acid sequence in the area of the C-terminal of the beta chain that was reproduced by swapping the proline and lysine residues at positions B28 and B29 to form insulin lispro.[9] This became available in the UK as Humalog in 1996. At the same time, Novo Nordisk were developing insulin aspart by replacing the proline residue at position B28 with aspartate,[10] and this was launched a few years later (Figure 7.3).

Insulin and glucose profiles

Insulin lispro

The initial studies of quick-acting insulin analogues confirmed that reducing self-aggregation led to a more physiological insulin curve when compared to human soluble insulin. A single sc injection of lispro insulin produced a rapid rise in the plasma insulin concentration within minutes to a higher peak and which then fell more rapidly (Figure 7.4).[11] Similar profiles were also obtained in patients with both Type 1 and Type 2 diabetes. These kinetic studies showed that the maximum concentration obtained with insulin lispro was around twice as high as equivalent doses of conventional human insulin and took around 60 minutes rather than 120 minutes to reach its maximum concentration. The analogue insulin was also almost completely absorbed after 4 hours.[12]

The glucose profiles observed following single injections of rapid-acting insulin analogues are also more physiological compared to those obtained with conventional insulins. Following injection, glucose starts to fall within 5 minutes, compared to the 30-40 minutes it takes for soluble insulin to reduce blood glucose. These differences compared to soluble insulin are also reflected in lower postprandial glucose concentrations following a test meal.[13] The potential effectiveness was also demonstrated by Heineman et al.,[10] who reported marked decreases in postpran-

(a)

(b)

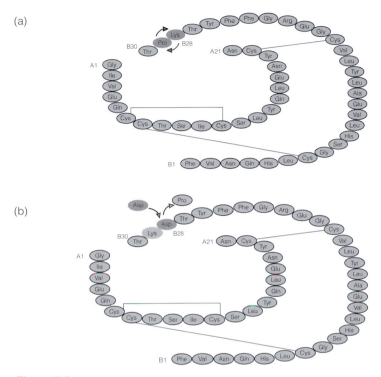

Figure 7.3

Physical structures of (a) insulin lispro and (b) insulin aspart.

dial hyperglycaemia in patients with Type 1 diabetes following a carbohydrate-rich test meal.

The insulin kinetic profile of insulin lispro also differs from human soluble insulin in other ways that may produce additional clinical benefits. Increasing doses of soluble insulin tends to increase the duration of action; however, this is generally not seen with insulin lispro in which the duration of action appears to be far less related to dose.[14] This might be useful in the treatment of patients needing large doses of insulin such as those with Type 2 diabetes. Furthermore, the altered onset of action according to injection site is far less prominent. ter Braak et al.[15] found that absorption rates of insulin lispro were similar from the arm, thigh and abdomen, in contrast to human soluble insulin that tends to be absorbed more rapidly from the abdomen and arm.

Insulin aspart

Similar effects on insulin and glucose profiles have also been demonstrated for insulin aspart. In one study, Lindholm et al.[16] also demonstrated that the pharmacokinetic effect of a quick-acting insulin analogue is greater than altering the timing of a premeal injection of soluble insulin

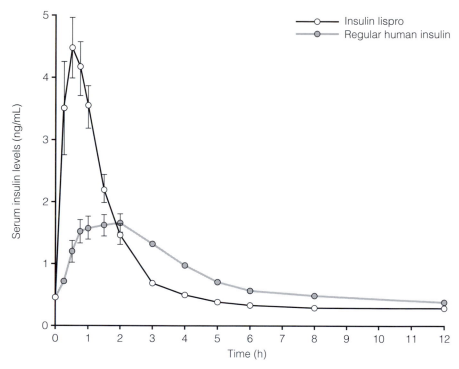

Figure 7.4

Serum insulin profiles of conventional soluble insulin and insulin lispro after a single
injection. Figure redrawn from Howey et al.[12]

(Figure 7.5). Although delaying the meal by 30–40 minutes produced
higher insulin concentrations at the time of eating compared to an injection given immediately preprandially, insulin levels after an injection of
insulin aspart given just before the meal were significantly higher. This
was reflected in the postprandial glucose concentrations, which were
significantly lower then those seen following injection of human soluble
insulin whatever the premeal interval (Figure 7.5).

The beneficial effects on postprandial glucose were initially demonstrated following a single injection of quick-acting insulin analogues, usually
before a comparable test meal. Studies examining 24-hour glucose profiles have confirmed the effect on postprandial glucose, as well as high-
lighting the potential limitations of quick-acting analogues. Home et al.[17]
measured 24-hour glucose profiles in patients with Type 1 diabetes who
were randomized to either premeal human soluble insulin or insulin
aspart as part of a basal bolus regimen with a single dose of isophane
(NPH) taken at bedtime. Postprandial glucose peaks were reduced at

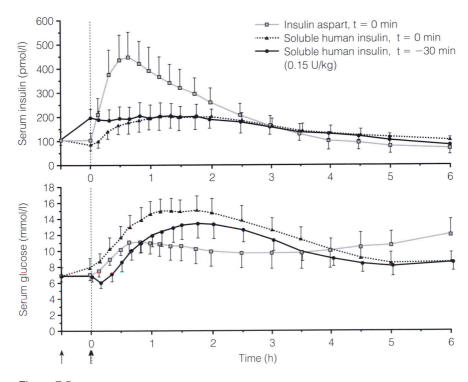

Figure 7.5

Serum insulin and glucose profiles after (a) a single injection and (b) test meal in patients with Type 1 diabetes. Figure redrawn from Lindholm et al.[16]

each of the three main meals but there was a tendency for the glucose concentration to rise between meals. The other striking difference when compared to human soluble insulin was a generally higher glucose concentration during the night. This was an early clue that insulin analogues might help to reduce the incidence of nocturnal hypoglycaemia.

In summary, the early studies of both quick-acting insulin analogues have confirmed the potential pharmacological benefits of more physiological insulin profiles. These also produce a lower postprandial and a higher overnight glucose, which might lead to significant clinical advantages.

Clinical trials

There has been a fairly extensive clinical trial programme studying the efficacy of both insulin lispro and insulin aspart. However, the usefulness of the data has often been limited by the requirement to satisfy the regulatory authorities, and to demonstrate safety and equivalence to existing agents rather than design high-quality studies to test clinical utility. This is demonstrated by the number of trials involving large patient numbers often with only moderate glycaemic control. It is unsurprising that the data from these studies provide limited information on clinical benefit. Furthermore, few studies have been blinded, raising concerns that at least some of the perceived benefit may be more to do with how much the new product has been 'sold' to patients rather than a true advance.[18] This is particularly true of outcomes that measure quality of life. It is noteworthy that one recent trial that used a double-blind design found few differences between conventional human soluble insulin and insulin lispro.[19] The predominance of open studies has been justified on the grounds that when taking human soluble insulin patients needed to leave a 30–45 minute gap to ensure maximum benefit, in contrast to rapid-acting insulin analogues that need to be injected immediately preprandially. However, as discussed above, the actual improvement in postprandial glucose values produced by waiting is marginal and may also increase the risk of hypoglycaemia as a result of a previous injection.[18] In practice, few patients consistently maintain a gap between injecting and eating as it is somewhat impractical.[20] Nevertheless, despite all of these limitations, a number of blinded studies have been undertaken and there are sufficient additional data from open studies to gain some idea of the clinical role of quick-acting analogues (Table 7.1).

Type 1 diabetes

Insulin lispro

Most large clinical trials have generally involved basal bolus regimens with one or two injections of isophane insulin as the basal insulin with insulin lispro compared to human soluble as the preprandial insulin using both parallel and crossover designs.

The main outcome measures have included glycaemic control, as measured by glycated haemoglobin HbA_{1c}, hypoglycaemia rates, home

Table 7.1 Indications for use of rapid-acting insulin analogues.

Strong evidence	Some evidence	Theoretical basis
Nocturnal hypoglycaemia in tightly controlled patients	Patient convenience	Selectively treating postprandial glucose in in Type 2 diabetes
Postprandial insulin in young children	Preprandial insulin in gestational diabetes	Missing snacks to lose weight
Continuous subcutaneous insulin infusion (CSII)	In Type 1 diabetes during pregnancy	

blood glucose profiles and various measures of quality of life. These large trials have demonstrated either relatively minor or no effect on glycaemic control.[21,22] Glucose profiles obtained during home blood glucose monitoring in many of the studies have demonstrated why improvement in overall glycaemic control has been relatively small, and has confirmed the results of 24 glucose profiles. The benefit of lower postprandial glucose is offset by the shorter duration of action, which leads to both a higher preprandial and fasting glucose. The shorter duration of action of analogues might be expected to reduce the risk of hypoglycaemia and this has been in confirmed in many of the trials. However, in most studies, there have been insufficient numbers of severe episodes to demonstrate a significant reduction (particularly as a severe episode was often defined as a coma or requiring glucagon). A meta-analysis has confirmed that lispro produces significant falls in the rates of severe hypoglycaemia but the reduction has been relatively modest.[23] The main effect appears to be upon nocturnal episodes; this reflects the tendency for human soluble insulin to accumulate during the day and contribute to high free insulin levels during the night. Reductions in both severe and nocturnal episodes have ranged from 10 to 25%. Unsurprisingly, it also appears that the largest falls in hypoglycaemia are seen in those at greatest risk; thus, patients undertaking intensive insulin therapy and exhibiting tight glycaemic control appear to have the greatest fall in hypoglycaemia. Holleman et al.[24] have demonstrated a 20% reduction in severe hypoglycaemic episodes (with a definition of severe hypoglycaemia that included external help). In an open study in which patients maintained particularly tight glycaemic control, with HbA_{1c} levels of c. 6.5% in both arms, a 60% fall in symptomatic nocturnal hypoglycaemic episodes was reported.[25]

Insulin aspart

The clinical trials involving insulin aspart have reported results similar to those for insulin lispro. Two large studies have recently been published, and interestingly, have both demonstrated a significantly lower HbA_{1c} level in those randomized to the quick-acting analogue.[26,27] However, the mean reduction of c. 0.2% has questionable clinical relevance. Those studies that have reported blood glucose profiles also show data very similar to those produced by insulin lispro with lower postprandial glucose values offset by higher post-absorptive concentrations. Rates of hypoglycaemia are lowered to a similar extent to those observed with insulin lispro. One recent study involving a crossover design of patients with tight glycaemic control and HbA_{1c} values of approximately 7.5% reported a 60% fall in major nocturnal hypoglycaemic episodes.[28]

The results of the large clinical trials involving both quick-acting insulin analogues have demonstrated rather modest clinical benefits, with either no or minor reductions in HbA$_{1c}$ levels compared to soluble insulin and relatively modest falls in rates of symptomatic hypoglycaemia, particularly at night. This is in part due to the nature of the study design, in which large number of patients are recruited to demonstrate both safety and efficacy. There is little incentive to tighten glycaemic control and the protocols that govern dose adjustment and basal insulin replacement are based on the pharmacokinetics of soluble insulin. In smaller studies, where the investigators have greater control over the protocol and other aspects of the trial, the benefits appear to be greater. This may involve the omission of between-meal snacks and dividing the basal insulin replacement into two injections given before breakfast and before bed. Perhaps the most successful demonstration of this approach was reported by Lalli et al.,[29] who gave individualized doses of NPH together with lispro insulin before each meal. They achieved extremely tight glucose control with relatively little hypoglycaemia (Figure 7.6), and were also able to demonstrate that physiological defences to hypoglycaemia were preserved. The approach was extremely labour intensive and it

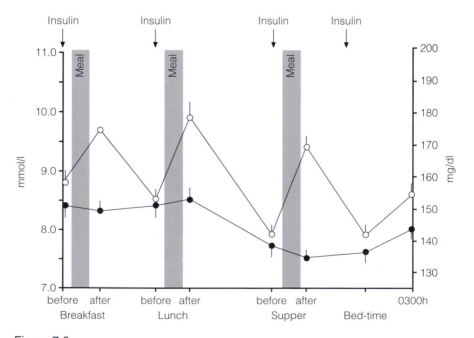

Figure 7.6

Home blood glucose monitoring in patients with Type 1 diabetes using either insulin lispro or soluble insulin and variable doses of NPH as mealtime insulin. ○ Hum-R ● lispro Taken from Lalli et al.[29]

seems unlikely that it could become routine clinical practice in busy units. However, the study demonstrates that different ways of using rapid-acting insulin analogues need to be developed if their clinical advantages are to be maximized.

Type 2 diabetes

Relatively few studies have reported the use of rapid-acting analogues in the management of Type 2 diabetes. This may in part be because few patients with Type 2 diabetes are currently treated with basal bolus regimens. One study has reported comparable glycaemic control and a slightly reduced rate of hypoglycaemic episodes in a group of 722 patients receiving insulin lispro.[22] In another, insulin lispro in combination with glibenclamide produced similar HbA_{1c} values to either a combination of evening NPH and glibenclamide or premeal soluble insulin and glibenclamide.[30] However, there is a lack of published data to indicate whether those with Type 2 diabetes who are intensively treated can achieve either tighter glycaemic control or less hypoglycaemia. One might anticipate that results would be similar to those with Type 1 diabetes.

However, there are other potential benefits that might result from the use of insulin analogues in people with Type 2 diabetes. There is increasing evidence that the excessive rise in postprandial glucose may have a disproportionate effect on both HbA_{1c} levels and cardiovascular risk. Such patients may, in time, benefit from treatment that specifically lowers postprandial glucose. Appropriate medication includes short-acting insulin secretagogues such as repaglinide or netaglinide. However, the rapid-acting insulin analogues, by replacing the deficient first phase insulin response, specifically reduce postprandial glucose values.[31] It remains unclear as to the best insulin regimens to use in patients with Type 2 diabetes, a question that was not answered by the UK Prospective Diabetes Study (UKPDS). However, the use of premeal rapid-acting insulin analogues has potential, particularly as it might allow such insulin-treated patients to safely miss snacks between meals, which in theory may limit weight gain. The ultimate benefit of such an approach will only be demonstrated by a fall in cardiovascular events following a controlled trial and results from such a study would not be available for some years. Nevertheless there seems merit in comparing preprandial insulin to more conventional insulin regimens using surrogate outcomes such as HbA_{1c} levels, weight and lipids.

The use of analogues in pre-mixed preparations

Many people with both Type 1 and Type 2 diabetes are treated with twice daily pre-mixed insulin as 70% isophane and 30% as human soluble.

Both Eli Lilly & Co and Novo Nordisk have developed mixtures of iso-phane and rapid-acting analogues of similar proportions. Mix 25 (Eli Lilly & Co) is now widely available and the Novo Nordisk preparation is likely to appear soon. These preparations lower postprandial glucose more effectively than mixtures containing human soluble insulin,[32] although this benefit obviously doesn't extend to the midday meal. However, giving the evening dose of isophane before the evening meal may make it difficult to lower fasting glucose levels on the following day without causing overnight hypoglycaemia. These limitations may explain in part why those treated with fixed-dose mixtures generally fail to achieve the tight levels of glycaemic control possible with basal bolus regimens. The results of ongoing clinical trials are required but to date the limited clinical trial evidence has failed to demonstrate a major benefit to patients. One study has compared the effect of pre-mixed insulin containing insulin lispro or human soluble insulin in similar proportions in 89 patients with Type 2 diabetes.[33] The authors reported a significant reduction in postprandial glucose with use of the insulin lispro mixture following a test meal, but fasting glucose levels were higher and there was no difference in gly-caemic control. The only demonstrable benefit to date of including a quick-acting insulin analogue with fixed-dose mixtures in standard pro-portions is the convenience of being able to inject immediately before the meal. However, since the clinical advantage of such a strategy has yet to be demonstrated, particularly in those with relatively poor metabolic con-trol, the evidence does not yet support switching patients to this type of preparation, particularly in view of the financial premium. More studies with tighter glucose targets are needed.

Rapid-acting analogues with continuous subcutaneous insulin infusion (CSII)

When CSII was originally introduced it was believed that such an approach could overcome the unfavourable pharmacokinetics of the available insulins, particularly, the longer acting preparations.[34] However, the results of clinical trials have not generally revealed major advantages, although minor falls in HbA_{1c} levels have been demonstrated. In the Dia-betes Control and Complications Trial (DCCT), those who chose pump therapy did not generally achieve either better glycaemic control or less hypoglycaemia. This finding is, at first sight, somewhat surprising but may reflect the tendency for self-association of conventional insulin which overcomes any benefit of constant basal insulin supply. This appears to be borne out by a study from Zinman et al.,[35] who randomized patients to CSII using either human soluble or insulin lispro in a double-blind crossover trial. HbA_{1c} levels were 0.3% lower while patients were taking insulin lispro and, although not significant, there was a trend for hypogly-caemic episodes to be lower on the analogue. These advantages have been confirmed in some,[36] but not all,[37] additional studies, although all have demonstrated the stability of quick-acting analogues when used in pumps.

Thus, the limited clinical trial data support the use of rapid-acting analogue insulin during CSII but the degree of benefit needs to be established by further trials.

Rapid-acting insulin analogues in children

Unsurprisingly, the pharmacokinetic advantages of rapid-acting analogues have also been demonstrated in children and adolescents with Type 1 diabetes,[38] but as yet there are few data to establish the clinical benefit in this group.

Rapid-acting insulin analogues may have a role in treating young children. Rapid-acting insulin analogues, when given postprandially, produce equivalent glucose control to a conventional soluble insulin given before the meal,[39,40] and the feasibility of such an approach in children under 5 years of age has also been reported.[41] The ability of parents to give an appropriate amount of insulin by calculating the dose after a child has eaten seems particularly useful for managing children whose eating patterns are irregular and is a robust indication for the use of rapid-acting insulin analogues. The place of insulin analogues in treating adolescents with diabetes is unclear. One study has shown the acceptability of lispro insulin in a group of relatively well-controlled teenagers, although the improved outcomes were confined to minor reductions in hypoglycaemia and patient acceptability.[42] Another study reported reductions in nocturnal hypoglycaemia but increased hypoglycaemia in the evening, prompting the authors to conclude that rapid-acting analogues should be combined with a different approach to between-meal snacks.[43] The shorter duration of action of rapid-acting analogues might, in theory, make those adolescents using them, and who regularly miss injections, more prone to diabetic ketoacidosis, although this has apparently not been observed in the few reported clinical trials. Whether it proves a problem in clinical practice remains to be seen.

Pregnancy

There is considerable potential in using insulin analogues in pregnancy. In those with Type 1 diabetes, glycaemic control is usually extremely tight and patients have to put up with a high risk of hypoglycaemia. It is anticipated that such a group would particularly benefit from reduced hypoglycaemia, although the increased tendency to ketosis suggests that twice daily NPH is probably the most appropriate choice of basal insulin. In gestational diabetes, postprandial glucose values predict fetal weight. Since in non-pregnant patients this is controlled more effectively with rapid-acting insulin analogues, they may be useful in the management of gestational diabetes. In one randomized trial, Jovanovic et al.[44] observed lower postprandial glucose in patients treated with insulin lispro in comparison with human soluble insulin but there was no difference in fetal outcome. They also demonstrated comparable anti-insulin antibody concentrations in the two groups and an absence of insulin lispro in cord blood.

However, there has been an understandable caution in using these agents where there have been questions raised about their safety, particularly as regards mitogenicity (see below). A letter detailing two congenital abnormalities in women using insulin lispro during pregnancy[45] has been followed by reassurance from larger series with normal outcomes. A further report of rapid progression of diabetic retinopathy in women using insulin lispro has been robustly challenged in a letter listing the other possible causes for such deterioration.[46] Unsurprisingly, neither of the manufacturers have made a formal trial in pregnancy an early priority. In the opinion of the present author, each case needs to be decided on its own merits, and both the clinician and patient should be involved in the decision. This is an area which would benefit considerably from a well-designed clinical trial, although reassurance will also be provided from an accumulation of clinical evidence.

Long-acting analogues

Two long-acting analogues, insulin glargine (produced by Aventis) and insulin detemir (produced by Novo Nordisk) are in an advanced stage of clinical development (Figure 7.7). Glargine is already on the market in the USA and Germany, and both preparations will presumably become generally available over the next few years.

Ironically, the currently available extended duration insulins were developed to save patients the necessity for repeated injections, before the concept of using exogenous insulin to mimic the physiology of the beta cell was developed. It is therefore not surprising that trying to use them to replace the basal insulin supply has generally been unsuccessful. Both isophane and lente insulins have a longer duration of action compared to soluble preparations but sc insulin produces insulin concentrations that peak some hours after injection.[47] Current long-acting preparations also exhibit marked inter- and intra-individual variability.[48] These limitations lead to a high risk of hypoglycaemia in tightly controlled patients, particularly at night. Various manipulations of timing and dose have been tried to overcome these problems but the lack of a suitable basal insulin is a major barrier to maintaining tight metabolic control with conventional preparations. The manipulation of the insulin molecule to produce a reliable basal insulin has involved two very different approaches.

(a)

(b)

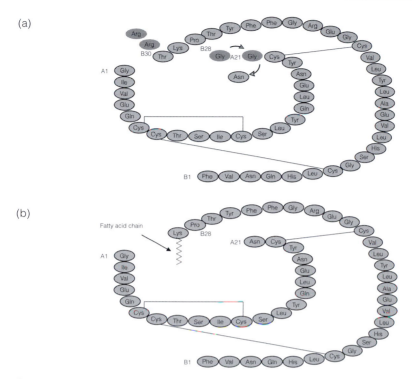

Figure 7.7

Physical structures of (a) insulin glargine and (b) insulin detemir.

Insulin glargine

Novo Nordisk were the first company to try and reduce the solubility of insulin by developing a preparation (NovoSol Basal) that was soluble at a slightly acid pH but which then precipitated in the more alkaline sc tissue.[49] However, its bioavailability was too low for clinical use. Hoechst (now part of Aventis) used the same principle in developing insulin glargine by adding two glycine residues to the alpha chain together with an extra arginine to the end of the beta chain to improve stability.[50] This insulin had much better bioavailability with a much flatter insulin profile than conventional extended action insulins (Figure 7.8).[51,52] Its increased solubility in the vial means that it is formulated as a clear preparation, which has the disadvantage of making it difficult to blind clinical trials.[53] It has been argued that such a property may reduce the intra-individual variability as there is no need for patients to resuspend the insulin in the vial before use,[54] but the data confirming this hypothesis have yet to appear. There are, as yet, insufficient data from clinical trials to come to any definite conclusions about its place in the management of diabetes.

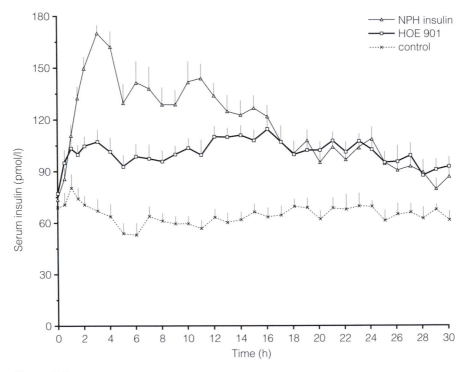

Figure 7.8

Serum insulin concentrations after subcutaneous injection of insulin glargine, NPH insulin and placebo in 15 normal subjects. Taken from Heninemann et al.[52]

Two recent trials involving a total of over 800 patients with Type 1 diabetes have compared insulin glargine to isophane insulin in a basal bolus regimen, demonstrating minimal falls in HbA_{1c} levels and slight but significant falls in rates of nocturnal hypoglycaemia.[55,56] Yki-Jarvinen et al.[57] studied 426 patients with Type 2 diabetes taking oral agents and either NPH or glargine at bedtime. Glycaemic control was tightened aggressively in both groups and symptomatic hypoglycaemia was lower in those receiving insulin glargine, particularly at night. Thus, the early data indicate that insulin glargine does not have a major effect on glycaemic control but can reduce hypoglycaemia.

Insulin Detemir

Novo Nordisk have used a different approach in developing their long-acting insulin analogue insulin detemir. They have modified the insulin molecule by attaching a fatty acid chain on the end of the beta chain, resulting in its binding to albumin.[58] Thus, the extended duration occurs due to its binding to albumin in sc tissue and its subsequently prolonged plasma half-life. Initial studies indicate that insulin detemir has a longer duration of action and lower intra-individual variability compared to NPH, but that its bioavailibility is lower.[59] Clinical trials are ongoing and have still to be published.

It is too soon to judge whether either of these long-acting insulin analogues will provide superior basal insulin replacement than current conventional extended duration preparations. The pharmacokinetics appear promising but the clinical trials involving the quick-acting insulin analogues have demonstrated that superior pharmacokinetic profiles do not necessarily predict major benefit in clinical trials. The early indications are that insulin glargine will reduce hypoglycaemia without major reductions in HbA_{1c} levels; there are not yet sufficient clinical data involving insulin detemir to make a judgement about it. However, as with the rapid-acting analogues, it may be that using them properly needs to be learnt before their effectiveness can be correctly assessed.

Safety

Mitogenicity

The mitogenic potential of the insulin preparation B10[Asp] has raised the question of the safety of insulin analogues. A number of attempts have been made to identify which of the features of a particular analogue are associated with mitogenic potential. Alterations in binding characteristics at both the insulin and IGF-1 receptor can promote cell growth although, since the affinity of natural insulin for the IFG-1 receptor is c. 1000 times lower, this receptor is not involved in the physiological actions of insulin.[60] However, it appears that both IGF-1 receptor affinity[61] and occupancy time of the insulin receptor[62] are associated with mitogenic effects in certain cell lines. Kurtzhals et al.[60] recently demonstrated that the mitogenic potential of different insulin analogues in an oesteosarcoma cell line was closely related to IGF-1 receptor affinity. Since insulin glargine had a six-fold greater affinity for the IGF-1 receptor, and greater mitogenic potency, the question of its safety was raised. However, the analogue B10[Asp], whose propensity to cause mammary tumours in vivo prompted its removal from clinical development, has a much higher occupancy time on the insulin receptor than insulin glargine does. Furthermore, other studies have not confirmed that insulin glargine has a high affinity for the IGF-1 receptor.[63,64] Thus the safety of insulin analogues, particularly glargine, remains unclear. In the present author's opinion, it seems reasonable to continue with the clinical evaluation of insulin glargine, particularly as it potentially offers significant clinical benefits. However, it is equally necessary to proceed cautiously and remain vigilant for any adverse effects. The issue of long- and medium-term safety has been raised,[65] and can only be definitely established by careful post-marketing surveillance.

Conclusions

The overwhelming evidence demonstrating the benefits of tight glycaemic control has resulted in more patients undertaking intensive insulin therapy, revealing the major limitations in conventional insulin therapy. Genetic engineering has produced two rapid-acting insulin analogues, insulin lispro and insulin aspart, with a reduced tendency to self-association. These exhibit more physiological insulin profiles after sc injection and reduce postprandial glucose when compared to conventional soluble insulin. However, clinical trials have revealed generally modest benefits with little or no improvement in HbA_{1c} levels and slight falls in hypoglycaemia. These rather disappointing results are partly due to the inability of regulatory trials to explore clinical benefit and also because it has taken time to learn how to use these preparations to their best advantage. However, it appears that the ability of rapid-acting insulin analogues to reduce nocturnal hypoglycaemia, particularly in those attempting to maintain tight glucose targets, is emerging as a robust indication for their use. Although their use in other circumstances is less well supported by trial data, it seems reasonable to evaluate the clinical benefit in individual cases. There are, as yet, insufficient data from clinical trials to determine the extent to which either of the new long-acting insulin analogues represent an important advance. It is possible that a combination of both quick- and long-acting analogues will prove able to maintain tight glycaemic control without being accompanied by severe hypoglycaemia, but the data are not yet available. Alternatively, such a desirable outcome may only prove possible by using completely different methods of insulin delivery.

References

1. The Diabetes Control and Complications Trial Group. The effect of intensive treatment of diabetes on the development and progression of long-term complications in insulin-dependent diabetes mellitus. New Engl J Med 1993; 329: 977–86.

2. Reichard P, Pihl M. Mortality and treatment side effects during long term intensive conventional insulin treatment in the Stockholm Diabetes Intervention Study. Diabetes 1994; 43:313–17.

3. Rizza RA, Gerich JE, Haymond MW, et al. Control of blood sugar in insulin-dependent diabetes: comparison of an artificial

endocrine pancreas, continuous subcutaneous insulin infusion and intensified conventional insulin therapy. New Engl J Med 1980; 303:1313–18.

4. Polonsky KS, Given BD, Van Cauter E. Twenty-four-hour profiles and pulsatile patterns of insulin secretion in normal and obese subjects. J Clin Invest 1988; 81: 442–8.

5. Blundell T, Dodson G, Hodgkin D, Mercola D. Insulin: the structure in crystal and its reflection in chemistry and biology. Adv Prot Chem 1972; 26:279–402.

6. Brange J, Ribel U, Hansen JF, et al. Monomeric insulins obtained by protein engineering and their medical implications. Nature 1988; 333:679–82.

7. Nielsen FS, Jorgensen LN, Ipsen M, et al. Long-term comparison of human insulin analogue B10Asp and soluble human insulin in IDDM patients on a basal/bolus insulin regimen. Diabetologia 1995; 38: 592–8.

8. Drejer K. The bioactivity of insulin analogues from in vitro receptor binding to in vivo glucose uptake. Diabetes Metab Rev 1992; 8: 259–85.

9. DiMarchi RD, Chance RE, Long HB, et al. Preparation of an insulin with improved pharmacokinetics relative to human insulin through consideration of structural homology with insulin- like growth factor I. Horm Res 1994; 41(Suppl 2): 93–6.

10. Heinemann L, Kapitza C, Starke AAR, Heise T. Time action profile of the insulin analogue B28Asp. Diabet Med 1996; 13:683–7.

11. Heinemann L, Starke AA, Heding L, et al. Action profiles of fast onset insulin analogues. Diabetologia 1990; 33: 384–6.

12. Howey DC, Bowsher RR, Brunelle RL, Woodworth JR. [Lys(B28), Pro(B29)]-human insulin. A rapidly absorbed analogue of human insulin. Diabetes 1994; 43: 396–402.

13. Tuominen JA, Karonen SL, Melamies L, et al. Exercise-induced hypoglycaemia in IDDM patients treated with a short- acting insulin analogue. Diabetologia 1995; 38:106–11.

14. Koivisto VA. The human insulin analogue insulin lispro. Ann Med 1998; 30:260–6.

15. ter Braak EW, Woodworth JR, Bianchi R, et al. Injection site effects on the pharmacokinetics and glucodynamics of insulin lispro and regular insulin. Diabetes Care 1996; 19:1437–40.

16. Lindholm A, McEwan J, Riis AP. Improved postprandial glycemic control with insulin aspart. Diabetes Care 1999; 22:801–5.

17. Home PD, Lindholm A, Hylleberg B, Round P. Improved glycemic control with insulin aspart. Diabetes Care 1998; 21:1904–9.

18. Berger M, Heinemann L. Are presently available insulin analogues clinically beneficial? Diabetologia 1997; 40(Suppl 2): S91–6.

19. Gale EAM. A randomized, controlled trial comparing insulin lispro with human soluble insulin in patients with Type 1 diabetes on intensified insulin therapy. Diabet Med 2000; 17:209–14.

20. Heinemann L. Do insulin-treated diabetic patients use an injection–meal-interval in daily life? Diabet Med 1995; 12:449–50.

21. Anderson JHJ, Brunelle RL, Koivisto VA, et al. Reduction of postprandial hyperglycemia and frequency of hypoglycemia in IDDM patients on insulin-analog treatment. Multicenter Insulin Lispro Study Group. Diabetes 1997; 46:265–70.

22. Anderson JHJ, Brunelle RL, Keo-

hane P, et al. Mealtime treatment with insulin analog improves postprandial hyperglycemia and hypoglycemia in patients with non-insulin-dependent diabetes mellitus. Arch Intern Med 1997; 157:1249–55.

23. Brunelle RL, Llewelyn J, Anderson JH, et al. Meta-analysis of the effect of insulin lispro on severe hypoglycemia in patients with Type 1 diabetes. Diabetes Care 1998; 21:1726–31.

24. Holleman F, Schmitt H, Rottiers R, et al. Reduced frequency of severe hypoglycemia and coma in well-controlled IDDM patients treated with insulin lispro. Diabetes Care 1997; 20:1827–32.

25. Heller SR, Amiel SA, Mansell P. Effect of the fast-acting insulin analog lispro on the risk of nocturnal hypoglycemia during intensified insulin therapy. Diabetes Care 1999; 22:1607–11.

26. Home PD, Lindholm A, Riist A. Insulin aspart vs human insulin in the management of long-term blood glucose control in Type 1 diabetes mellitus: a randomized controlled trial. Diabet Med 2000; 17:762–70.

27. Raskin P, Guthrie RA, Leiter L, et al. Use of insulin aspart, a fast-acting insulin analog, as the mealtime insulin in the management of patients with Type 1 diabetes. Diabetes Care 2000; 23:583–8.

28. Heller SR, Colagiuri S, Vaaler S, et al. Reduced hypoglycemia with insulin aspart: a double-blind, randomised, crossover trial in Type 1 diabetic patients. Diabetes (in press).

29. Lalli C, Ciofetta M, Del Sindaco P, et al. Long-term intensive treatment of Type 1 diabetes with the short-acting insulin analog lispro in variable combination with NPH insulin at mealtimes. Diabetes Care 1999; 22:468–77.

30. Bastyr 3rd EJ, Johnson ME, Trautmann ME, et al. Insulin lispro in the treatment of patients with Type 2 diabetes mellitus after oral agent failure. Clin Ther 1999; 21: 1703–14.

31. Bruttomesso D, Pianta A, Mari A, et al. Restoration of early rise in plasma insulin levels improves the glucose tolerance of Type 2 diabetic patients. Diabetes 1999; 48: 99–105.

32. Koivisto VA, Tuominen JA, Ebeling P. Lispro Mix25 insulin as premeal therapy in Type 2 diabetic patients. Diabetes Care 1999; 22:459–62.

33. Roach P, Yue L, Arora V. Improved postprandial glycemic control during treatment with Humalog Mix25, a novel protamine-based insulin lispro formulation. Humalog Mix25 Study Group. Diabetes Care 1999; 22:1258–61.

34. Pickup JC, Keen H, Parsons JA, Alberti KG. Continuous subcutaneous insulin infusion: an approach to achieving normoglycaemia. Br Med J 1978; 1:204–7.

35. Zinman B, Tildesley H, Chiasson JL, et al. Insulin lispro in CSII: results of a double-blind crossover study. Diabetes 1997; 46:440–3.

36. Melki V, Renard E, Lassmann-Vague V, et al. Improvement of HbA1c and blood glucose stability in IDDM patients treated with lispro insulin analog in external pumps. Diabetes Care 1998; 21:977–82.

37. Renner R, Pfutzner A, Trautmann M, et al. Use of insulin lispro in continuous subcutaneous insulin infusion treatment. Results of a multicenter trial. German Humalog-CSII Study Group. Diabetes Care 1999; 22:784–8.

38. Mortensen HB, Lindholm A, Olsen BS, Hylleberg B. Rapid appearance and onset of action of insulin aspart in paediatric subjects with

Type 1 diabetes. Eur J Pediat 2000; 159:483–8.

39. Schernthaner G, Wein W, Sandholzer K, et al. Postprandial insulin lispro. A new therapeutic option for Type 1 diabetic patients. Diabetes Care 1998; 21:570–3.

40. Brunner GA, Hirschberger S, Sendlhofer G, et al. Post-prandial administration of the insulin analogue insulin aspart in patients with Type 1 diabetes mellitus. Diabet Med 2000; 17:371–5.

41. Rutledge KS, Chase HP, Klingensmith GJ, et al. Effectiveness of postprandial Humalog in toddlers with diabetes. Pediatrics 1997; 100:968–72.

42. Grey M, Boland EA, Tamborlane WV. Use of lispro insulin and quality of life in adolescents on intensive therapy. Diabetes Educat 1999; 25:934–41.

43. Mohn A, Matyka KA, Harris DA, et al. Lispro or regular insulin for multiple injection therapy in adolescence. Differences in free insulin and glucose levels overnight. Diabetes Care 1999; 22:27–32.

44. Jovanovic L, Ilic S, Pettitt DJ, et al. Metabolic and immunologic effects of insulin lispro in gestational diabetes. Diabetes Care 1999; 22:1422–7.

45. Diamond T, Kormas N. Possible adverse fetal effect of insulin lispro. New Engl J Med 1997; 337:1009; discussion 1010.

46. Jovanovic L. Retinopathy risk: what is responsible? Hormones, hyperglycemia, or Humalog?: response to Kitzmiller et al. Diabetes Care 1999; 22:846–8.

47. Heinemann L, Richter B. Clinical pharmacology of human insulin. Diabetes Care 1993; 16(Suppl 3): 90–100.

48. Lauritzen T, Pramming S, Gale EA, et al. Absorption of isophane (NPH) insulin and its clinical impli-cations. Br Med J (Clin Res Ed) 1982; 285:159–62.

49. Jorgensen S, Vaag A, Langkjaer L, et al. NovoSol Basal: pharmacokinetics of a novel soluble long acting insulin analogue. Br Med J 1989; 299:415–19.

50. Brange J, Volund A. Insulin analogs with improved pharmacokinetic profiles. Adv Drug Deliv Rev 1999; 35:307–35.

51. Lepore M, Pampanelli S, Fanelli C, et al. Pharmacokinetics and pharmacodynamics of subcutaneous injection of long-acting human insulin analog glargine, NPH insulin, and ultralente human insulin and continuous subcutaneous infusion of insulin lispro. Diabetes 2000; 49:2142–8.

52. Heinemann L, Linkeschova R, Rave K, et al. Time-action profile of the long-acting insulin analog glargine (HOE 901) in comparison with those of NPH insulin and placebo. Diabetes Care 2000; 23:644–9.

53. Vajo Z, Duckworth WC. Genetically engineered insulin analogs: diabetes in the new millenium. Pharmac Rev 2000; 52:1–9.

54. Bolli GB, Owens DR. Insulin glargine. Lancet 2000; 356:443–5.

55. Ratner RE, Hirsch IB, Neifing JL, et al. Less hypoglycemia with insulin glargine in intensive insulin therapy for Type 1 diabetes. US Study Group of Insulin Glargine in Type 1 Diabetes. Diabetes Care 2000; 23:639–43.

56. Pieber TR, Eugene-Jolchine I, Derobert E. Efficacy and safety of HOE 901 versus NPH insulin in patients with Type 1 diabetes. The European Study Group of HOE 901 in Type 1 diabetes. Diabetes Care 2000; 23:157–62.

57. Yki-Jarvinen H, Dressler A, Ziemen M. Less nocturnal hypoglycemia and better post-dinner glucose control with bedtime insulin

glargine compared with bedtime NPH insulin during insulin combination therapy in Type 2 diabetes. HOE 901/3002 Study Group. Diabetes Care 2000; 23:1130–6.

58. Kurtzhals P, Havelund S, Jonassen I, et al. Albumin binding of insulins acylated with fatty acids: characterization of the ligand–protein interaction and correlation between binding affinity and timing of the insulin effect in vivo. Biochem J 1995; 312:725–31.

59. Brunner GA, Sendhofer G, Wutte A, et al. Pharmacokinetic and pharmacodynamic properties of long-acting insulin analogue NN304 in comparison to NPH insulin in humans. Expl Clin Endocr Diabetes 2000; 108:100–5.

60. Kurtzhals P, Schaffer L, Sorensen A, et al. Correlations of receptor binding and metabolic and mitogenic potencies of insulin analogs designed for clinical use. Diabetes 2000; 49:999–1005.

61. Slieker LJ, Brooke GS, DiMarchi RD, et al. Modifications in the B10 and B26–30 regions of the B chain of human insulin alter affinity for the human IGF-I receptor more than for the insulin receptor. Diabetologia 1997; 40(Suppl 2): S54–61.

62. Hansen BF, Danielsen GM, Drejer K, et al. Sustained signalling from the insulin receptor after stimulation with insulin analogues exhibiting increased mitogenic potency. Biochem J 1996; 315:271–9.

63. Bahr M, Kolter T, Seipke G, Eckel J. Growth promoting and metabolic activity of the human insulin analogue [GlyA21,ArgB31, ArgB32]insulin (HOE 901) in muscle cells. Eur J Pharmac 1997; 320:259–65.

64. Berti L, Kellerer M, Bossenmaier B, et al. The long acting human insulin analog HOE 901: characteristics of insulin signalling in comparison to Asp(B10) and regular insulin. Horm Metab Res 1998; 30:123–9.

65. Buse J. Insulin glargine (HOE 901): first responsibilities: understanding the data and ensuring safety. Diabetes Care 2000; 23: 576–8.

8
Erectile dysfunction: a highly treatable condition?

William D Alexander

Introduction

Erectile dysfunction (ED), or impotence, may be defined as the inability to obtain or sustain an erection sufficient for sexual satisfaction. It is a common and often distressing problem that can significantly affect the quality of life of diabetic men and their partners. In recent years effective treatments have become more accessible and more acceptable, particularly with the availability of orally active therapy. More men are therefore likely to ask for help and ED should now be considered highly treatable by diabetes teams in both primary and secondary care. This review considers the management of this important problem.

Historical perspectives

In the past most men with ED who attended physicians would have been labelled as having psychological problems, told they would have to accept the problem and dismissed as suffering from the natural process of ageing. This was not totally unreasonable because effective treatment was largely unavailable.

Physical treatments for ED have been sought and attempted for many centuries by a few enthusiasts but the medical profession has not really taken the problem very seriously until the last two decades.

In the nineteenth century, and before, apart from the contribution of witchcraft and religion, useless suggestions might include rest and abstention. More aggressive practitioners might consider flagellation, massage or galvanic stimulation. The early twentieth century saw the beginning of the first vacuum tumescence devices and various splints. Some surgical techniques were also explored. Many aids also became, and remain, available from sex shops, magazines and catalogues, and although not expensive they are relatively ineffective for men with severe ED as occurs in diabetes. The situation changed dramatically in the

1970s with the publication, by Masters and Johnson,[1] of Human sexual inadequacy, which drew attention to sexual problems and particularly to psychological treatments. This approach, although helpful generally, did not solve the problems of men with a physical cause, as is usually the case in diabetes.

Subsequently, advances in penile prostheses made available the possibility of an effective surgical treatment. The pioneering work of Virag[2] and Brindley,[3] on the use of intracavernosal injections of vasoactive drugs, then produced a further major advance, which stimulated increasing interest in the importance of ED as a potentially treatable condition and revolutionized treatment availability. This interest also raised the profile of vacuum devices that became more formally available and effective. The public then became more aware of treatments and requests to the medical profession increased. This demand and the treatment advances then led to the development of ED management as a significant clinical specialty. Research and development, largely by urologists, rapidly led to greater understanding of the pathophysiology, management and treatment. There did however remain significant inhibitions amongst the public and physicians, and it was only in the 1990s that treatment availability really became a practical reality for most diabetic men. The recent development of effective oral therapy has now made the management of ED possible as a routine part of diabetic clinical practice both in primary and secondary care.

Pathophysiology

Erection is predominantly a neurovascular event under psychological, hormonal and autonomic nervous system control. Hormonal factors are particularly relevant to libido and arousal. The penile tissues involved in erection itself include the corpora cavernosa that contains blood vessels and interconnected sinusoidal spaces. These erectile structures are innervated by autonomic nerves that are influenced by higher centres involved during sexual arousal and activity. Flaccidity is maintained by increased sympathetic tone and erection produced by the parasympathetic. Neurotransmitters released by the parasympathetic induce smooth muscle relaxation and subsequent increased arteriolar vasodilatation and expansion of the sinusoidal spaces. If the blood flow is sufficient, erection occurs and as the pressure rises so the veins draining the sinusoidal spaces become occluded. Adequate smooth muscle relaxation and blood flow is essential for a firm erection to occur, and an effective veno-occlusive mechanism is then essential for maintenance of erection. After ejaculation the process is reversed and flaccidity restored by increasing sympathetic nervous system activation.

ED may occur with dysfunction of any of these mechanisms, including both psychological and physical components. In diabetes, ED is usually due to a physical cause, although there may be superimposed secondary psychological factors including the performance anxiety that occurs in association with the experience of failure. Traditionally, ED has been thought to be directly related to the neuropathic or vascular complications of diabetes.[4] Recent interest has been focused on the structure and function of the endothelium and smooth muscle of the corpora cavernosa themselves, which may exhibit degeneration and endothelial dysfunction related to advanced glycation products adversely affecting the activated nitric oxide pathway.[5-6] ED is probably multifactorial in origin and a precise cause often difficult to identify. Clinically, this is not that important, and in practice treatment options and preferences are determined by personal choice rather than likely aetiology.

Prevalence and the relationship between erectile dysfunction (ED) and diabetes

ED is one of the commonest complications to affect diabetic men. Mild degrees may affect > 75% some of the time and 35% may suffer from persistent problems. The prevalence increases with age and > 60% of men over the age of 60 will be affected.[7] It is most common in Type 2 diabetes because of the age of the patients, and associated cardiovascular disorders, risk factors and multiple drug regimes. ED may precede, or occur at any time after, the diagnosis of diabetes. In Type 1 diabetes, ED is related, like many other complications, to the duration of diabetes, the degree of metabolic control and the presence of other risk factors.

Diabetes is a chronic metabolic disorder with many complications and associated factors that predispose to erectile dysfunction. These include:

- psychological stresses of living with a chronic disease;
- metabolic effects of hyperglycaemia and excessive protein glycosylation;
- penile disorders: balanitis, phimosis, Peyronie's disease;
- premature ageing and degeneration of corpora cavernosal smooth muscle and endothelial function;
- microvascular disease;
- sensory and autonomic neuropathy;
- macrovascular disease and its risk factors, including dyslipidaemia and its treatment;
- hypertension and antihypertensive drug regimes.

Increasingly, intensive management of cardiovascular risk factors is being recommended both for primary and secondary prevention of cardiovascular events. In particular, this relates to the ever lower targets of blood pressures and normalization of the blood lipid profile. In order to achieve such targets, increasing numbers of diabetic patients are required to take multiple antihypertensive drugs regimes and lipid-lowering agents. Most blood-pressure-lowering agents, if effective, are associated with ED and the increasing intensity of such regimes is likely to increase the prevalence of ED even more. This needs to be borne in mind when starting such treatments and the problem openly discussed to try and maximize compliance.

Men with diabetes are also not exempt from the ravages of smoking and excessive alcohol.

Screening and awareness regarding erectile dysfunction (ED) and its treatment

Despite increased publicity regarding ED there remains general embarrassment and a lack of understanding about the nature of the condition, and the availability and suitability of treatments.[8] This is a pity because one or other of the treatment options is likely to be successful, and successful treatment can reverse the negative effect that ED can have upon the quality of life and self-esteem of the man who suffers from the condition.[7]

Direct questioning regarding ED could, or maybe should, be part of the routine annual review of the diabetic male, whether it be in primary care or hospital clinic. ED is common, it affects quality of life, is easily identified and there are effective treatments, provided that the service is prepared to make them available. Furthermore, identification of ED may be important as the first overt sign of serious underlying cardiovascular disease that requires investigation and treatment in its own right.

An alternative to direct questioning or male health questionnaire at annual review is to ensure there are awareness posters and leaflets available at all diabetic clinics so men and/or their partners can avail themselves of information without necessarily having to discuss the problem when unprepared (Figure 8.1).

Whichever approach is taken, it is surely important that it is ensured that diabetic men no longer suffer in silence, or without at least the chance to discuss and try treatment if they so wish. The gains that can be achieved from resolution of the problem of ED make the management of this condition rewarding for both the patient and the health-care professional.

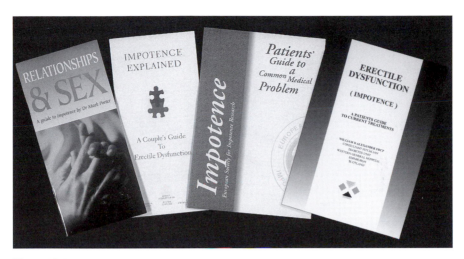

Figure 8.1
Some examples of ED information leaflets.

Assessment and investigation

A past inhibiting factor, apart from embarrassment, to the provision of treatment was the suggested need for complex assessments and investigations that appeared to be outside the time available and the expertise of the non-specialist. This should no longer be the case because no complex investigations are required, and there is now a consensus on the minimal requirements for the assessment and investigation of ED. One example of such a consensus document is that produced by the Erectile Dysfunction Alliance (EDA) and produced by a multidisciplinary group of experts in the field.[9]

The objective of a consultation is to obtain an idea of likely aetiologies, to further investigate and treat them as necessary, and also to agree a management plan to include an assessment of contra-indications, explanation and instruction on the use of the various treatment options.

History

History and examination are the mainstay of assessment. It may be most appropriate for a specific consultation time to be arranged rather than trying to fit it into a busy general diabetic clinic. A reasonably relaxed atmosphere and attitude is more likely to help men overcome any embarrassment they may have. It is preferable for the partner to be present and men should be invited to bring them with them, but this is not always possible or appropriate and should not be insisted upon.

The history should be sufficient to provide an answer to the following questions:

- what exactly is the problem?;
- what is the likely cause?;
- what is the partner's attitude?;
- what treatments is the man aware of, and what has he tried and how?;
- how much of a problem is it and what would he like done about it?

A drug history is important, including the relevance of alcohol, tobacco and any other recreational agents. Many therapeutic drugs have been implicated.[10] In the context of diabetes, perhaps the most important are the antihypertensive agents. The UK Prospective Diabetes Study (UKPDS) group has shown significant benefits regarding morbidity and mortality with tight blood pressure control, and that this will often require the use of multiple agents.[11] This is likely not only to increase the prevalence of ED but also to reduce the opportunities to discontinue offending drugs. It is unlikely that any regime can be sufficiently altered such as to improve ED without unacceptable loss of blood pressure control. Anyway, in the present author's experience, unless there is a specific temporal association between the onset of ED and a specific drug, there is not much benefit to be had by altering antihypertensive regimes. A further important aspect of a drug history is to avoid potentially dangerous interactions with proposed treatments for the ED (e.g. nitrates and Viagra; anticoagulants and vacuum devices).

Examination and investigation

Examination and investigation are important not only in relation to the ED but also to detect and further assess other conditions that may require treatment in their own right. Examination of the genitalia is essential to detect primary penile abnormalities such as balanitis, phimosis, penile curvature and fibrosis from Peyronie's disease, or congenital or traumatic conditions. Such abnormalities may require referral for surgical correction prior to embarking upon treatment for the ED.

Examination is also important in assessing the practicality of physical treatments such as injection or vacuum therapy, e.g. there may be difficulties in men with a very large abdomen and a small penis. Some treatments also require good manual dexterity.

In the context of a diabetes clinic, it is likely that men will already have had a neurological and full cardiovascular assessment. This is clearly of importance because cardiovascular disease is so commonly an accompaniment, and its management is essential to prevent morbidity and mortality.

Endocrine investigation is recommended, particularly in men who present with loss of libido or show signs of hypogonadism, and might include blood tests to assess thyroid function together with testosterone, luteinising hormone/follicle-stimulating hormone and prolactin. Primary hypogonadism or hypogonadism secondary to occult pituitary tumours or disease, although rare, are important conditions not to miss.

No further investigations are considered essential unless indicated by specific system findings from the history and examination.

Other common problems associated with erectile failure are:

- loss of libido: this may be due to psychological problems or be a presenting feature of hypogonadism. It may also occur as a phenomenon secondary to the experience of sexual failure;
- balanitis and phimosis: this may be painful or unpleasant and deter from sexual activity. Antifungal treatment or circumcision may be required. A tight phimosis can become very painful or split on restoration of erection if this has not occurred for many years;
- Peyronie's disease may require referral for correction if the curvature is painful and/or so great as to prevent satisfactory penetration;
- retrograde or failed ejaculation: this may occur in association with autonomic neuropathy. Tricyclic drugs may be helpful for retrograde ejaculation. The main implication of these disorders relates to infertility and the man may require referral for specialist techniques of sperm retrieval;
- premature or quick ejaculation: current treatments include local anaesthetic creams, selective serotonin reuptake inhibitors or physical treatments for ED that may prolong the duration of erection.

Treatment of erectile dysfunction (ED)

Men who seek advice are those whose erectile function is insufficient to allow them to reliably enjoy satisfactory sexual activity. In men with diabetes this is usually predominantly a physical rather than psychological problem. There may be associated psychological factors, particularly related to performance anxiety as a result of having experienced failure, and there may also be relationship problems that require further discussion.

A physical cause is suggested if:
- the onset was gradual;
- erectile failure is complete;
- it occurs regardless of the circumstances;
- there are no overt psychological factors;
- there is an identifiable physical cause.

Conversely, a psychological cause might be suggested if:
- the onset was sudden without obvious explainable physical cause, e.g. trauma, drugs, etc.;
- it varies according to the circumstances;
- there are overt psychological factors;
- there is no clear physical cause.

Men with diabetes and ED will therefore usually require a physical treatment. One or other of such available treatments is likely to be very effective and currently includes:

- oral sildenafil (e.g. Viagra);
- intracavernosal self-injection treatment;
- intraurethral therapy;
- vacuum devices;
- surgical insertion of penile prostheses.

General counselling

Whatever further treatment is to be agreed, general counselling is important. This should include an explanation of ED, its prevalence and likely causes. It is helpful to men and their partners for their problem to be put into perspective. A discussion should always include reference to the partner, be they present or not, and to the relationship. The implications of treatments should be covered.

It may also be helpful, particularly if there has been performance anxiety, to discuss techniques such as the Masters and Johnson sensate focusing exercises that may help communication and understanding between partners, and thereby improve sexual relationships.

Men with general psychological problems and a likely psychological cause for their ED should be referred for psychosexual therapy, if they are agreeable and it is available. The presence of associated psychological problems should not exclude the use of physical treatments – the two should be considered as complimentary to each other.

Physical treatments

Whichever treatment is to be used as first choice it is generally agreed that all options should be discussed. Giving the man a leaflet regarding ED and its treatment may also be helpful, which then enables him to share information with his partner.

Sildenafil citrate (Viagra) – an oral agent

The arrival of an effective oral agent such as sildenafil has not only made treatments more available and acceptable to men with ED but has also enabled much treatment to be initiated in primary care and not be restricted to limited hospital specialist resources. Sildenafil is currently the treatment of first choice for most men with ED.

Sildenafil is a phosphodiesterase-5 (PDE5) inhibitor – its action is illustrated in Figure 8.2. With sexual arousal, nerve impulses are transmitted along so-called nonadrenergic, noncholinergic (NANC) nerves and nitric oxide synthase (NOS) is activated, releasing NO. In the penis this produces smooth muscle relaxation around the blood vessels in the corpora

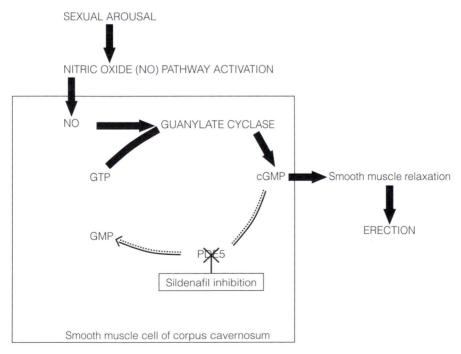

Figure 8.2

Schematic representation of action of sildenafil on phosphodiesterase-5 (PDE5) and cyclic guanosine monophosphate (cGMP) in smooth muscle cell of corpora cavernosum. GTP, guanosine 5'-triphosphate; GMP, guanosine 5'-phosphate.

cavernosal and trabecular network, and an erection is produced by the marked increase in blood flow. The relaxation mechanism activated by NO involves guanylate cyclase and cyclic guanosine monophosphate (cGMP). cGMP is hydrolysed by the enzyme PDE5. In ED there is reduced cGMP in the tissues and its normal hydrolysis by PDE5 limits its availability further. The effect of sildenafil is therefore to increase the availability of cGMP by inhibiting PDE5, thereby reducing cGMP clearance. Its action will not be effective in the absence of activation of the NO pathway, which is dependent upon sexual arousal (unlike self-injection therapy that can produce an erection under any circumstances).

Sildenafil can be expected to be effective in c. 60% of diabetic men, the majority (> 90%) requiring a dose of 100mg. These figures relate mainly to men with Type 2 diabetes, many with cardiovascular disease.[12] It is equally effective in Type 1 diabetes but there is insufficient evidence available to know whether the effectiveness is different in the two types of diabetes and, for example, in the presence of neuropathy versus vascular disease or risk factors.

It is important that men understand its actions in order to ensure effective use. Sildenafil has an onset of action of 20–60 minutes, absorption being quickest if taken on an empty stomach.

Sildenafil should be given a reasonable trial prior to abandoning it as ineffective. Initially there may be superimposed problems of performance anxiety, particularly in men with longstanding ED and/or particuarly high expectations. A suggested reasonable trial would be to initially prescribe 4 × 50mg tablets: 50mg can be tried on two separate occasions and if these were ineffective then the remaining 2 × 50mg should be taken together (i.e. 100mg). Subsequently, a prescription for 4 × 100mg tablets should be provided. Should these not be effective then other methods of treatment should be considered. It is not recommended to use doses > 100mg.

Side effects of Sildenafil
Side effects are uncommon, usually only mild and seldom lead to discontinuation of treatment. They include headache, dyspepsia and flushing. Transient colour visual disturbance may occasionally occur due to the retinal effects of PDE6 inhibition. Diabetic retinopathy need not be considered a contraindication.

Sildenafil and nitrates
The concomitant use of sildenafil and nitrates is absolutely contraindicated because of the risk of potentially serious hypotension. This also applies to other NO donors such as nicorandil. Nitrates, although usually used for the symptomatic treatment of angina, may be used as recreational drugs or occasionally as patches or creams for phlebitis. They may also be used in hospital to enhance venous access. It is clearly important not only to be sure sildenafil is not prescribed while people

take nitrates, but also that men have not taken sildenafil within the previous 24 hours if they present to emergency medicine departments with symptoms that might require nitrate prescribing. In this circumstance nitrates should be used very cautiously and with careful blood pressure monitoring.

Managing ED in men taking nitrates for angina

It is not an uncommon situation for a man with ED and diabetes to be taking multiple drugs for secondary cardiovascular protection, and these may include nitrates in either short- or long-acting forms. Nitrates are a symptomatic treatment for angina and are not of prognostic significance. Consideration should therefore be given to discontinuing the nitrate rather than immediately excluding the possibility of sildenafil treatment for the ED. Sildenafil is safe in men with cardiovascular disease (see below). Prescribed nitrates may be seldom used and a legacy of past angina. A careful history will reveal whether they are a necessity. If not, and the man is not suffering significant exercise-induced angina, then a trial without nitrates can be considered. Short-acting nitrates should not be used within 24 hours of sildenafil and long-acting ones within 1 week, and vice versa. Men using 'as required' short-acting nitrates should be made aware of this and warned that on no account should they use their nitrate preparation. If long-acting nitrates are being taken these can be discontinued and if there is no problem with angina after 1 week then sildenafil can be prescribed. Should angina be troublesome during the week then an alternative anti-anginal therapy can be used such as a calcium-channel blocker.

Cardiovascular risk, ED and sildenafil

Initially, following the release of sildenafil for clinical use, there was concern expressed regarding sildenafil's cardiovascular safety. Despite reassurances from the results of more recent surveillance and published studies, and guidance, some doctors remain concerned and are reluctant to prescribe sildenafil to men with multiple vascular risk factors or overt cardiovascular disease. This is unreasonably overcautious. The initial clinical trials showed a rate of serious cardiovascular events of 4.1 per 100 man years of treatment compared with 5.7 per 100 man years for placebo. Subsequent studies in men with severe coronary artery disease detected no adverse cardiovascular effects.[13–14]

The other relevant issue is whether it is safe for men with cardiovascular disease to resume sexual activity at all. This may be a more important issue than whether it is safe to take sildenafil. The physiological stress of sexual activity is no more than that of most normal daily activities and is similar to walking at a normal pace for 20 minutes.[15] Sexual intercourse is the possible cause of a myocardial infarct (MI) in < 1% of cases. The risk of a MI in non-cardiac patients is about 1 in 1,000,000 during daily life and 2.5 in 1,000,000 in the 2 hours immediately after sexual intercourse.

In the cardiac patient these figures rise to 10 in 1,000,000 and 30 in 1,000,000, respectively, but this is a very low absolute risk.[16] If there is concern from the man or his partner, as may the case after a recent MI, a 6 minutes exercise test using the Bruce protocol will be physiologically similar to sexual activity. Many men will be taking beta blockers anyway and these will further reduce any effect of sexual activity on pulse rate and blood pressure.

The most important aspect of this consideration is the assessment of the cardiac status per se. If there is sufficient concern about the safety of sexual activity then there is anyway a need for formal cardiac assessment in its own right. High-risk cardiac patients with refractory/unstable angina or severe heart failure should be assessed by a specialist cardiologist. Sexual activity and treatments for ED, including sildenafil, should also probably be avoided within 14 days of a stroke or MI.

Consensus statements have now been published both in the UK and USA, and both have concluded that sildenafil can be safely used in men with stable cardiovascular disease.[17,18] Such advice applies to all current treatments for ED.

Other oral and topical agents

Many other drugs have been studied and these include the following: the oral agents yohimbine, phentolamine, apomorphine, bromocriptine, trazodone and topical nitrates, minoxidil, and alprostadil. Evidence for effectiveness in severe organic ED as occurs in diabetic men, has been disappointing. New PDE inhibitors of proven efficacy are currently under development and should become available within the next 2 years.

Intraurethral therapy

Intraurethral alprostadil has been developed as an alternative to injection therapy. Drugs may be absorbed through the epithelium of the urethra and gain access to the smooth muscle of the corpora cavernosa via the spongiosal and corpora cavernosal veins.

The medicated urethral system for erection (MUSE) is a system that delivers a pellet of prostaglandin E_1 (PGE1) into the urethra (Figure 8.3). The patient should first lubricate the urethra by micturating. The stem of the device is then inserted fully into the urethra and a pellet delivered by pressing the button on the end of the device. It is recommended then that the man remains standing and massages the penis for c. 10 minutes. Although there was considerable initial enthusiasm and success,[19] subsequent experience has been disappointing,[20,21] particularly in men with severe ED as occurs in diabetes.

The dose of PGE1 is high, ranging from 250 to 1000µg, and penile pain may occur. Pain may also be experienced in the thighs, presumably due to more peripheral spread of the PGE1.

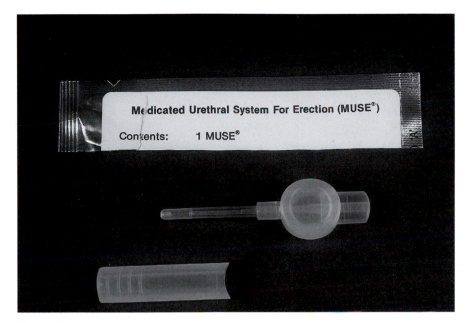

Figure 8.3
Medicated urethral system for erection (MUSE).

Intracavernosal injection therapy

Intracavernosal self-injection with vasoactive drugs is one of the major second-line treatments for ED and can be highly effective, and relatively simple and painless to administer. Its advantages include broad efficacy, safety and rapidity of action.

It involves the injection of a small (< 1ml) volume of a vasoactive drug into one of the corpora cavernosa using either a syringe or an injector device with needle sizes similar to those used for the injection of insulin. The technique is simple but it is essential that men are carefully instructed on its use, by the doctor or nurse, to be sure that they are going to be competent, safe and confident enough to use it themselves at home. This advice should be reinforced by written and pictorial instructions (Figures 8.4 and 8.5).

The foreskin should be retracted and the penis stretched by pulling the glans with one hand. The injection is given into the side of the penis avoiding the glans and any obvious superficial veins (Figure 8.6). Care should also be taken to avoid the deep midline veins on the dorsum of the penis and the urethra ventrally.

The erection may take 10 minutes to occur and last from 15 minutes to several hours. Detumescence may not occur after ejaculation and men should be aware of this. The current drug of choice is PGE1 (alprostadil). This is available either in packs with syringes, needles, and separate vials of powder and diluent to be mixed (e.g. Viridal or Caverject), or with simpler injector devices and dual chamber vials (e.g. Caverject Dual Chamber or Viridal Duo) (Figures 8.4 and 8.7). Currently, Caverject Dual Chamber is the simplest to instruct and use. Preparations are available in different dosage packs; very high doses require separate mixing.

Other agents include papaverine, phentolamine, and combined phentolamine and vasoactive intestinal peptide (VIP), although availability is variable. Combinations, unlicensed in the UK, can be used for men not responding to conventional doses of PGE1 (> 40µg).

Side effects include bruising, painful erection, penile scarring and the potential for a prolonged erection (> 4 hours) that requires emergency medical detumescence. The latter is dose related and can be largely prevented by careful dosing instructions.

Dosage should be determined by the man in the normal environment of his own home and not at a clinic visit. He should be given instructions to start with a small dose and gradually increase on separate occasions until the lowest effective dose is found. Written advice on incremental dose increases should be provided.

Recommended doses of drugs for intracavernosal injection:

Alprostadil: Starting dose 5-10µg;
                incremental increases by 5µg up to 20µg;
                                       10µg up to 40µg;
                consider combination drugs if requirement > 40µg.

Papaverine: Starting dose   10mg;
                incremental increases   5mg up to 20mg;
                                       10mg up to 60mg.

Combinations should start with combinations of minimum doses and increase by similar increments to those above. Combinations may also include phentolamine or VIP.

The combination of phentolamine and VIP can be particularly useful in men who do not respond to, or who experience pain with PGE1. Its main side effect is facial flushing but this is usually short lived. It is produced commercially in a simple autoinjector device as Invicorp but availability has been unreliable.

Should a prolonged erection occur (> 4 hours), the man should attend for emergency treatment, be it day or night, to prevent irreversible hypoxic damage to the penis. Simple manoeuvres such as ice packs or vigorous leg exercise can be tried initially. He should be given written instructions on what to do in the event of this rare complication. These instructions should be taken with him to a casualty department in case they are unfamiliar with the procedure.

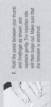
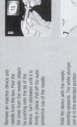

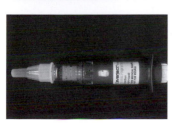

Figure 8.4

Intracavernosal injection treatment: Caverject dual chamber device and schematic representation.

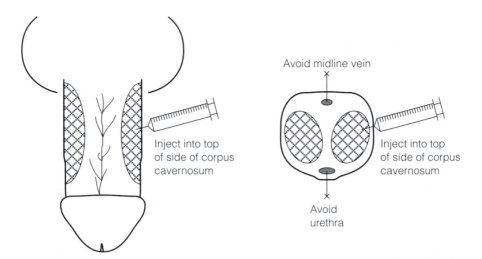

Figure 8.5

Intracavernosal injection treatment: Schematic representation.

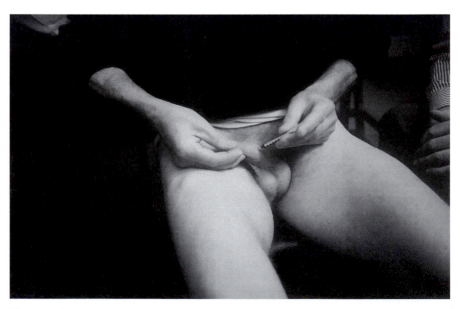

Figure 8.6

Intracavernosal injection treatment: a patient injecting.

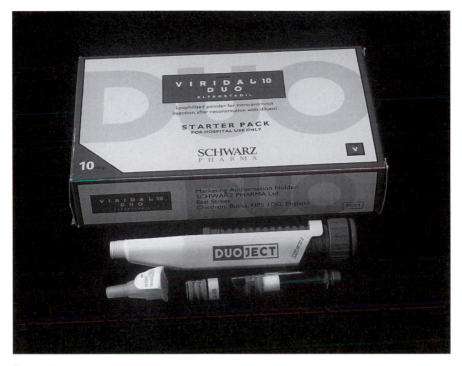

Figure 8.7

Intracavernosal injection treatment: Viridal Duo injector device.

Suggested treatment procedure for prolonged erection:
(1) a 25gauge butterfly is inserted into one of the corpora;
(2) aspirate 50ml of blood and apply pressure for 5 minutes;
(3) aspirate a further 50ml if (2) fails, irrigate with heparinized saline and again apply pressure;
(4) if (3) fails, inject 200µg of phenylephrine – repeat if (4) fails;
(5) if all measures fail, surgical treatment will be required.

Injection therapy is not contraindicated in men taking anticoagulants though extra care is required to prevent excessive bruising.

Intracavernosal injection therapy revolutionized the treatment of ED in the 1980s but is now usually a second-line treatment to sildenafil, unless the latter is contraindicated. A number of other compounds are under investigation. These—combination therapy and new simple injection devices—may further increase efficacy, acceptability and reduce unwanted side effects.

Vacuum Erection Devices (Figure 8.8)

There are now many different devices available but the principle is similar in all of them. The equipment consists of a clear plastic cylinder, a vacuum pump and a constriction ring. The cylinder and pump are assembled and the constriction ring mounted on the open end of the cylinder. The cylinder is placed over the penis and held tight against the pubis – some lubrication is required. The vacuum pump is then operated and when the penis is firm enough the constriction ring is slipped off the cylinder and around the base of the penis. This should produce an erectile state sufficient for intercourse. The constriction ring should not be left in place for > 30 minutes.

Vacuum devices are available by mail order from various manufacturers and most will supply an instruction video. Careful instruction and practice is important for success. They should be successful in up to 70% of men, regardless of the aetiology and severity of the ED. They are most successful in men with longstanding and understanding partners. They may not be so suitable for the single man embarking upon new relationships, as they may appear rather cumbersome and intrusive.

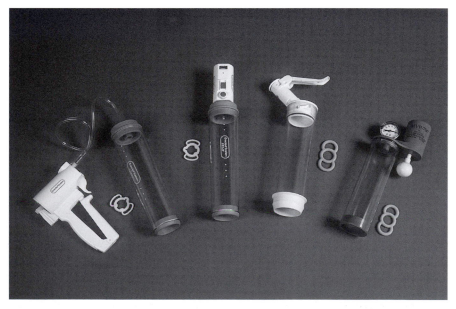

Figure 8.8
Examples of some vacuum tumescence devices.

Complications include discomfort, bruising and ejaculatory block. Extreme caution is required if patients are taking anticoagulants.

Vacuum devices can be used in combination with other treatments, including being used as an adjunct to penile prostheses or for men whose prostheses have had to be removed.

These devices cost from £100–300 and this may be one of the inhibiting factors to many men. Order forms and explanatory leaflets are available from the manufacturing companies and a supply should be kept in all diabetes centres or surgeries providing a diabetes care service.

Surgical treatment with penile prostheses

Now that there is such successful medical treatment it is only a small minority of men who will require, or wish to proceed to, surgical insertion of a penile prosthesis.

Some indications for surgical treatment might include:

* congenital or acquired anatomical abnormalities, e.g. micropenis;
* severe corporal fibrosis: post-injection therapy, Peyronie's disease, etc.;
* failure of other treatments;
* patient preference and unwillingness to try, or persevere with, other treatments.

Penile prostheses may either be of the semi-rigid or inflatable type. With proper patient selection and an experienced surgeon the success rate is high. It is a permanent solution, provided that there are no complications or mechanical failures, and may be considered a primary option in younger men with total and irreversible ED who do not respond well to oral therapy.

Conclusions

ED is common amongst diabetic men. It is usually organic and the cause multifactorial. Diabetic men with ED respond well to most medical treatments. Sildenafil is usually safe to use for men with multiple vascular risk factors, multiple drug regimes or overt cardiovascular disease. The management of this important condition should be a routine part of diabetes care. This management should at least include the assessment and investigation of, and treatment with, oral agents and/or vacuum devices.

Intracavernosal self-injection is a simple technique and at least one member of the diabetes care team should develop expertise in its instruction and provision. Referral to surgical specialists should now be reserved for men requiring surgical treatments such as penile prostheses.

References

1. Masters WH, Johnson VE. Human sexual inadequacy. Churchill: London; 1970.

2. Virag R. Intracavernous injection of papaverine for erectile failure. Lancet 1982; 2:938.

3. Brindley GS. Cavernosal alpha-blockade: a new treatment for investigating and treating erectile impotence. Br J Psychol 1983; 143:332–7.

4. Veves A, Webster L, Chen TF, et al. Aetiopathogenesis and management of impotence in diabetic males: 4 years experience from a combined clinic. Diabet Med 1995; 12:77–82.

5. Saenz de Tejada I, Goldstein I, Azadzoi K, et al. Impaired neurogenic and endothelium-mediated relaxation of penile smooth muscle from diabetic men with impotence. New Engl J Med 1989; 320: 1025–30.

6. Padma-Nathan H, Cheung D, Perelman N, et al. The effects of ageing, diabetes and vascular ischaemia on the biochemical composition of collagen found in the corpora and tunica of potent and impotent men. Int J Impot Res 1990; 2(Suppl 2):75–6.

7. Price D, O'Malley BP, James MA, et al. Why are impotent diabetic men not being treated. Prac Diabetes 1991; 8:10–11.

8. Cummings MH, Meeking D, Warburton F, Alexander WD. The diabetic male's perception of erectile dysfunction. Prac Diabetes Int 1997; 14:100–2.

9. Ralph D, McNicholas T, for the Erectile Dysfunction Alliance. UK management guidelines for erectile dysfunction. Br Med J 2000; 321:499–503.

10. Parkinson M, Bateman N. Disorders of sexual function caused by drugs. Prescribers J 1994; 34: 183–9.

11. UK Prospective Diabetes Study Group. Tight blood pressure control and risk of macrovascular and microvascular complications in Type 2 diabetes:UKPDS 38. Br Med J 1998; 317:703–13.

12. Rendell MS, Rajfer J, Wicker PA, Smith MD, for the Sildenafil Diabetes Study Group. Sildenafil for treatment of erectile dysfunction in men with diabetes. J Am Med Ass 1999; 281:421–6.

13. Conti CR, Pepine CJ, Sweeney M. Efficacy and safety of sildenafil citrate in the treatment of erectile dysfunction in patients with ischemic heart disease. Am J Cardiol 1999; 83:29C–34C.

14. Hermann HC, Chang G, Klugherz BD, Mahoney PD. Hemodynamic effects of sildenafil in men with severe coronary artery disease. New Engl J Med 2000; 342: 1622–6.

15. Bohlen JG, Held JP, Sanderson MO, et al. Heart rate, rate pressure product, and oxygen uptake during four sexual activities. Arch Intern Med 1984; 144:1745–8.

16. Müller JE, Mittleman A, Maclure M, et al. Triggering myocardial infarction by sexual activity. Low absolute risk and prevention by regular physical exertion. Determi-

nants of Myocardial Infarction Onset Study Investigators. J Am Med Ass 1996; 275:1405–9.

17. Jackson G, Betteridge J, Dean J, et al. A systematic approach to erectile dysfunction in the cardio-vascular patient: a consensus statement. Int J Clin Prac 1999; 53:445–51.

18. Cheitlin MD, Hunter AM Jr, Brindis RG, et al. Use of sildenafil (Viagra) in patients with cardiovascular disease. Circulation 1999; 99:168–77.

19. Padma-Nathan H, Hellstrom WJ, Kaiser FE, et al. Treatment of men with erectile dysfunction with transurethral alprostadil. Med-

icated Urethral System for Erection (MUSE) study group. New Engl J Med 1997; 336:1–7.

20. Shabsigh R, Padma-Nathan H, Git-tleman M, et al. Intracavernous alprostadil alfadex is more effica-cious, better tolerated, and pre-ferred over intraurethral alprostadil plus optional actis: a comparative, randomized, crossover, multicentre study. Urology 2000; 55:109–13.

21. Fulgham PF, Cochrane JS, Den-man JL, et al. Disappointing results with transurethral alpro-stadil in men with erectile dysfunc-tion. J Urol 1998; 159(Suppl): 905A.

9

What new therapies are there for the treatment of diabetic neuropathy?

Aristidis Veves, Antonella Caselli and Panayiotis A Economides

Introduction

Diabetic neuropathy has been defined by the Consensus Conference of San Antonio as a peripheral neuropathy, either clinically evident or sub-clinical, that occurs in the setting of diabetes mellitus without other causes.[1] It is one of the most common long-term complications of diabetes mellitus and is clinically present in 30–50% of all diabetic patients.[2–3] It should also be remembered that diabetic neuropathy is not a single entity but, rather, a variety of syndromes that may be encountered either in isolation or in combination, causing considerable morbidity and mortality. Numerous attempts at classifications have been made and one scheme, based on clinical features, firstly proposed by Boulton and Veves, is summarized in Table 9.1.[4]

Despite numerous efforts over the last two decades, none of the tested therapeutic approaches has yet been approved for clinical use and at present good glycemic control is the only available strategy to prevent

Table 9.1 Classification of diabetic neuropathy.

Somatic		Autonomic
Polyneuropathies	Mononeuropathies	
Sensorimotor	Isolated	Cardiovascular
Proximal motor	Cranial	Gastrointestinal
Truncal	Truncal	Genitourinary
	Multiple	Miscellaneous

185

the development of the disease. The lack of a complete understanding of the pathogenic mechanisms underlying nerve damage, the difficulty in extrapolating data from animal studies to the human situation and the availability of only surrogate measures of nerve function may be some of the reasons for this failure. Nevertheless, a variety of experimental studies have provided new insights into the pathogenesis of the disease and new therapeutic approaches are currently under investigation and, hopefully, will be proven successful in the near future.

This chapter will include an overview of the main clinical features and the new concepts in the pathogenesis and diagnosis of the disorder, with a special focus on the new therapies that are currently under consideration.

Clinical features

The most common type of diabetic neuropathy is the distal symmetric polyneuropathy. This type of neuropathy is probably the most important one, as it plays a major role in the development of foot ulceration, the leading cause of hospitalization in diabetic patients and of non-traumatic amputation in developed countries.[5] The distal symmetric polyneuropathy is both sensory and motor, involving small myelinated and unmyelinated fibers and large myelinated fibers.[6] It is characterized by an insidious onset and a progressive development, initially involving the most distal parts of the lower extremities and then spreading proximally. The most common symptoms that patients complain of are numbness and a sensation of walking on cotton, paresthesias, dysesthesias, and neuropathic pain, described as a burning sensation, a sharp stabbing pain or a deep aching feeling. Nocturnal exacerbation of symptoms is quite characteristic. However, it is important to emphasize that most of the patients are asymptomatic and can reach the final stages of the disease, i.e. foot ulceration, without any symptoms. Therefore, the absence of symptoms does not necessarily mean the absence of diabetic neuropathy.

The main clinical signs are reduced or absent sensation to pain, touch and temperature in a 'stocking-and-glove' distribution, loss of vibration and proprioceptive sensation, and absent ankle reflexes. Motor involvement results in muscle weakness and atrophy. Wasting of the intrinsic muscles of the foot causes the prominence of the metatarsal heads and climbing toes, resulting in high plantar pressures. The loss of the protective sensitivity combined to foot structural and functional abnormalities represent the main causative factors in the development of callus and foot ulceration.[7-9]

Another less common diabetic polyneuropathy is proximal motor neuropathy. The main features of this syndrome are atrophy and weakness of the thigh muscles, often associated with troublesome pain and/or sensory loss. This is an acute polyneuropathy and full recovery over 6–12 months is the rule.

In addition to the polyneuropathies, diabetic patients are also susceptible to a variety of mononeuropathies. Amongst cranial nerve lesions, the third nerve is the most commonly affected. Intermittent chest or abdominal pain in a nerve root distribution characterizes thoracolumbar neuropathy/radiculopathy. Limb neuropathies include radial, median, ulnar and peroneal nerve palsies. The etiology of mononeuropathies is unknown and they are usually reversible within 3–6 months.

Involvement of the autonomic nervous system is a serious and often overlooked component of diabetic neuropathy and it usually correlates with the presence of peripheral somatic neuropathy.[10] It is associated with a higher risk of sudden death and a considerable reduction in life expectancy.[11] Autonomic impairment can involve any system of the body and its major manifestations are cardiovascular, gastrointestinal and genitourinary. Parasympathetic denervation is responsible for nocturnal hypertension, gastroparesis, and bladder and erectile dysfunctions, while orthostatic hypotension and retrograde ejaculation are related to sympathetic denervation. Reduced or absent variation of heart rhythm, silent myocardial infarction and sudden death are the most severe consequences of cardiovascular autonomic neuropathy.

Pathogenesis

Although the disease process is relatively well described, there is still uncertainty regarding the mechanisms that lead to nerve dysfunction in diabetes. In the past, two pathogenic hypotheses have been proposed: the metabolic hypothesis and the hypoxic one.[12,13] According to the metabolic hypothesis, hyperglycemia, through activation of the polyol pathway, leads to an increase in intracellular sorbitol that, in turn, causes low myoinositol levels and reduced Na^+–K^+-ATPase activity, which are responsible for the nerve damage. On the other hand, according to the hypoxic hypothesis, diabetes is responsible for microcirculation impairment that leads to nerve blood flow impairment, resulting in endoneurial hypoxia and nerve degeneration.[14]

It is currently apparent that the metabolic and vascular pathways are linked, and that both contribute to the development of the syndrome (Figure 9.1). More specifically, endothelial dysfunction has been suggested as the common denominator between metabolic abnormalities and impaired nerve blood flow, and therefore, as the pivotal factor in the development of diabetic neuropathy.[15] Abnormal endothelial function has been described not only in patients with established diabetic neuropathy but also in the earlier stages of the disease.[16,17] The impaired synthesis and/or function of nitric oxide (NO), the main vasodilator released by the

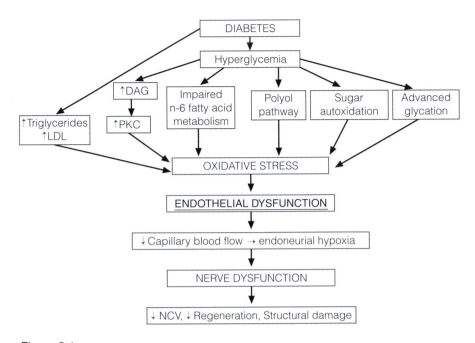

Figure 9.1

New concepts in the pathogenesis of diabetic neuropathy.
DAG, diacylglycerol; LDL, low density lipoprotein–cholesterol; NCV, nerve conduction velocity; PKC, protein kinase C.

endothelium, are believed to determine microvascular insufficiency, endoneurial hypoxia and nerve dysfunction.[18]

Many glucose-related metabolic pathways can cause endothelium dysfunction: e.g. increased aldose reductase activity leading to: an imbalance in nicotinamide adenine dinucleotide phosphate (NADP)– reduced NADP (NADPH); auto-oxidation of glucose leading to the formation of reactive oxygen species (ROS); advanced glycation end-products (AGE) produced by non-enzymatic glycation of proteins; abnormal n6 fatty acid metabolism; and inappropriate activation of protein kinase C.

Other factors can also contribute to the development of diabetic neuropathy and are under investigation at present. These include mitochondrial dysfunction of dorsal root ganglia, aberrant monofilament phosphorylation and disruption in the production of nerve growth factors, namely nerve growth factor (NGF), neurotrophin-3 (NT-3), brain-derived neurotrophic factor (BNDF) and neurotrophin 4/5 (NT-4). Thus, the prevailing concept today is that neuropathy is the final result of various pathways and does not have a single cause.

Diagnosis

The diagnosis of diabetic neuropathy should be based on clinical symptoms, clinical signs, quantitative sensory testing, electrophysiological tests and sural nerve biopsies. The clinical signs can be tested using simple equipment, such as a pin to test pain perception, cotton wool to test touch perception and a tuning fork to test vibration perception. Vibration perception can be also quantified using a biothesiometer and a vibration perception threshold (VPT) of 25V or more is able to identify patients at high risk of foot ulceration.[7] An even simpler method is the Semmes Weinstein Monofilament (SWM): a 5.07 monofilament is able to apply a force of 10g on a skin region and patients who cannot feel this pressure are at high risk of foot ulceration. In a recent prospective trial, the presence of clinical signs and/or the insensitivity to a 5.07 SWM had a sensitivity of 99% in predicting foot ulceration.[19]

Electrophysiology and sural nerve biopsies are the most accurate methods to diagnose and quantify diabetic neuropathy, but are recommended only for the conduction of clinical research. A major disadvantage of both these techniques is that they only test the function of large nerve fibers, which represent 25% of the peripheral nerve. Recently, a new technique that allows the study of small fibers has been developed.[20] It relies on the quantification of the epidermal nerve fibers by immunostaining and, as it requires only a skin-punch biopsy, it is a relatively easy, reproducible and reliable technique.[21,22]

An alternative technique to evaluate quantitatively the C nociceptive fiber function is through the measurement of the nerve axon reflex. The stimulus of the C nociceptive nerve fibers travels not only in the orthodromic direction, towards the spinal cord, but also antidromically, stimulating adjacent C fibers that secrete a number of vasomodulators, such as substance P and histamine, and cause local vasodilatation. This short circuit, or nerve axon reflex, is responsible of the Lewis' triple flare response to injury. Recent studies from the present authors have shown that the nerve axon reflex-mediated vasodilation accounts for approximately one third of the total endothelium-dependent vasodilation and, as expected, it is markedly reduced in presence of diabetic peripheral neuropathy.[23] The assessment of this hyperemic response may represent a new method to evaluate the C fibers' function in diabetic patients and it might be used as an objective end-point measurement of sensory deficit in clinical trials.

Finally, it should also be remembered that there is no single test that is pathognomonic of the disease, so that the diagnosis of diabetic neuropathy is one of exclusion. Some of the most common causes that should be excluded before the diagnosis is made are alcohol abuse, medications, vitamin B_{12} deficiency, uremia and spinal disorders.

Treatment

As previously mentioned, diabetic neuropathy is a progressively deteriorating disorder characterized by a complex and multifactorial etiopathogenesis. Therefore, its treatment should be based upon the underlying pathogenic mechanisms that lead to nerve damage rather than on symptoms. The possible interventions at the level of each proposed mechanism are summarized in Figure 9.2.

Metabolic control

Persistent hyperglycemia is the primary factor in the pathogenic cascade leading to diabetic neuropathy. Although knowledge was initially based on small observational studies, significant progress has been made over the last decade with the completion of two large prospective trials, the Diabetes Control and Complications Trial (DCCT) that involved Type 1 diabetic patients and the UK Prospective Diabetes Study (UKPDS) that involved Type 2 patients.[24–28] The DCCT enrolled 1441 Type 1 diabetic patients who were randomized to conventional and intensive insulin treatment. This study proved that a glycated hemoglobin (HbA$_{1c}$) reduction

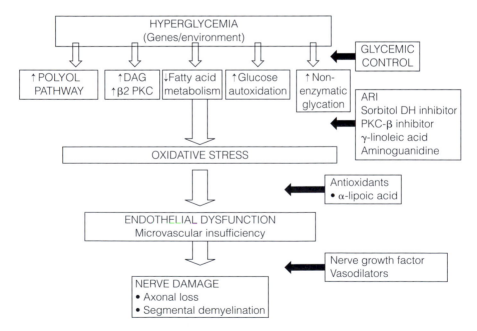

Figure 9.2

Pathogenesis and therapy of diabetic neuropathy.

from 9 to 7% for a mean follow-up of 6.5 years was able both to reduce the onset of diabetic neuropathy (from 9.6 to 2.8%) and to slow its progression.[25,26] The UKPDS enrolled 3867 newly diagnosed Type 2 diabetic patients and followed them for a mean period of 10 years.[27] Although the effect of intensive treatment on the incidence of microvascular complications was a secondary end-point of this study, a 1% reduction in mean HbA$_{1c}$ was associated with a reduction in risk of 37% for microvascular complications.[28]

Both of these studies showed the absence of a threshold of glycemia below which risk of diabetic neuropathy no longer decreased, emphasizing the importance of achieving glycemic levels as close as possible to the nondiabetic range.[29] However, euglycemia is only able to halt the progression, rather than reverse it, once the nerve damage has established. This can best be seen in patients who achieved euglycemia by pancreas transplantation: 2–3 years after transplantation, the nerve deterioration stabilized but nerve function never came back to normal levels.[30]

Aldose Reductase Inhibitors (ARI)

Increased polyol pathway activity has long been considered the main pathogenic mechanism leading to the development of diabetic neuropathy. More specifically, it was initially suggested that increased intracellular glucose levels resulted in increased sorbitol levels through the action of the aldose reductase enzyme. Therefore, it seemed reasonable at the time to suggest that inhibition of the aldose reductase enzyme should be expected to prevent diabetic neuropathy, or at least halt its progression.[31]

It has been more than 20 years since the first aldose reductase inhibitor (ARI), alrestatin, was found to prevent sorbitol accumulation in the nerve of diabetic and galactosemic rats. A large number of clinical trials with more than 30 different compounds have been conducted since then, but there is still no conclusive evidence regarding the efficacy of these compounds (Table 9.2). A possible reason for this may be the poor design of early ARI studies: the main limits of these trials are the small sample sizes, the short length (usually < 12 months), and the absence of reproducible and standardized methods to assess nerve function.[32]

Tolrestat was the first ARI to be licensed for the treatment of diabetic neuropathy in certain countries, although it was subsequently withdrawn due to serious side effects. A meta-analysis of three large randomized clinical trials,[33] including 738 patients with a treatment duration of 24–52 weeks, showed that tolrestat significantly reduced the development of motor nerve loss compared with placebo (> 40%), and the magnitude of the benefit was c. 1m/s.

Over the last 2-3 years, encouraging results have been reported with zenarestat, a new ARI that achieves a very satisfactory inhibition of nerve

Table 9.2 Aldose reductase inhibitor (ARI) trials in human neuropathy.

Authors	Design[a]	Duration of active treatment	Results[a]
Alrestatin			
Culebras 1981[85]	uncntr	5 days	Symptomatic improvement
Handelsman 1981[86]	sb, nonrmd, co	4 months	Symptomatic improvement
Fagious 1981[87]	db, rmd	12 weeks	Improvement of symptoms, VPT and ulnar mcv
Sorbinil			
Judzewitsch 1983[88]	db, rmd	9 weeks	Improvement of peroneal mcv and median mcv and scv
Jaspan 1983[89]	sb	3–5 weeks	Symptomatic improvement
Young 1983[90]	db, rmd, co	4 weeks	Improvement of symptoms and sural sap
Lewin 1984[91]	db, rmd, co	4 weeks	No improvement
Fagious 1985[92]	db, rmd	6 months	Improvement of posterior tibial mcv and ulnar nerve F, wl and dsl
O'Hare 1988[93]	db, rmd	12 months	No benefit
Guy 1988[94]	db, rmd	12 months	No benefit
Sima 1988[95]	db, rmd	12 months	Improvement of symptoms, sural sap and mfd
Ponalrestat			
Ziegler 1991[96]	db, rmd	12 months	No benefit
Krentz 1992[97]	db, rmd	12 months	No benefit
Tolrestat			
Ryder 1986[98]	db, rmd	8 weeks	Improvement of median mcv
Boulton 1990[99]	db, rmd	12 months	Improvement of paraesthetic symptoms and peroneal mcv
Macleod 1992[100]	db, rmd	6 months	Improvement of VPT, median and ulnar mcv
Boulton 1992[101]	db, rmd, withdrawal	12 months	Improvement of symptoms, median and peroneal mcv
Giugliano 1993[102]	db, rmd	12 months	Improvement of autonomic measurements and VPT
Giugliano 1995[103]	db, rmd	12 months	Improvement of autonomic measurements and VPT
Zenarestat			
Green 1999[34]	db, rmd	52 weeks	Improvement of peroneal and sural cv and small unmyelinated fiber density

*sb, single blind; db, double blind; uncntr, uncontrolled; nonrmd, nonrandomized; rmd, randomized; co, crossover; mcv, motor nerve conduction velocity; scv, sensory nerve conduction velocity; sap, sensory action potential; wl, wave latency; dsl, distal sensory latency; VPT, vibration perception threshold; mfd, myelinated fibre density.

aldose reductase. The results of a 52-week, randomized, placebo-controlled, multiple-dose, clinical trial that enrolled a large number of diabetic patients with mild to moderate peripheral polyneuropathy, have recently been published.[34] The two primary efficacy end-points were nerve conduction velocity (NCV) changes in sural, median and peroneal nerves and sural myelinated nerve fiber density (MFD) changes. The measurement of nerve sorbitol content was used to provide evidence of a satisfactory polyol pathway inhibition. Both the sensory and motor NCV declined in the placebo group, while a dose-dependent improvement in the zenarestat-treated group was observed. Total MFD tended to decrease in the placebo and low-dose treatment groups, and to increase in the high-dose groups, but these differences were not statistically significant. Furthermore, a selective dose-dependent effect on the small nerve fibers was reported. Despite these encouraging results, zenarestat was also withdrawn because of serious adverse effects.

Epalrestat is another ARI that has been approved in Japan for clinical use. A post-market analysis, which included more than 5000 patients with diabetic neuropathy, recently reported an improvement of motor and sensory nerve conduction velocities and vibration threshold.[35] In addition, a small open-label, nonrandomized, non-placebo-controlled clinical trial showed that epalrestat treatment induced a significant regeneration of small dermal nerve fibers.[36] Finally, fidarestat is another new ARI currently under investigation. Preliminary results in experimental diabetes have demonstrated sufficient suppression of sorbitol accumulation, and prevention of functional and structural nerve changes.[37,38]

Thus, despite intensive efforts over the last two decades, there has been a failure to convincingly show clinical efficacy of the ARI and introduce them to clinical practice. The use of new more potent compounds that are powerful enzyme inhibitors and are devoid of serious side effects may prove more efficacious compared to the previously tested compounds, but this remains to be verified.

New insights in the action of ARI

Over the last several years, it has been realized that ARI may also act through other pathways and that it is possible that their efficacy is related to this additional activity. Thus, the oxidation of NADPH to NADP by the enzyme aldose reductase can limit NO synthesis by cofactor competition, since NADPH is an obligate cofactor for nitric oxide synthase as well. Furthermore, NADPH oxidation impairs the glutathione (GSH) redox cycle, which is an important cellular protection against oxygen free radicals. ARI can therefore have an antioxidant action. Animal studies have shown that ARI prevent the development of impaired NO-mediated, endothelium-dependent relaxation in large vessels, and that NO inhibitors completely block the beneficial actions of ARI on nerve conduction velocity and nerve blood flow.[39–41]

ARI can also reduce the intracellular formation of AGE. A significant reduction in the levels of Nε-(carboxymethyl)lysine (CML) and other glycation precursors were observed in the erythrocytes of diabetic patients after a 2-month treatment with epalrestat and these changes were significantly related to the reduction in the erythrocyte sorbitol or fructose contents.[42] The rate of formation of CML and other glycoxidation products is considered to be dependent on the level of oxidative stress, and the reduction in the oxidative stress secondary to ARI treatment can, in part, explain the findings of this recent study. Finally, ARI can be related to NGF production. In recent studies in experimental diabetes, ARI treatment improved the decreased content of NGF in the sciatic nerves of diabetic rats.[43]

Sorbitol Dehydrogenase Inhibitors

The role of the second half of the polyol pathway, i.e. the conversion of sorbitol to fructose, in the development of diabetic neuropathy has also been investigated over the last few years. The oxidation of sorbitol to fructose by sorbitol dehydrogenase with reduction of NAD^+ to NADH was initially proposed to cause a state of hyperglycemic pseudohypoxia, which can be involved in the development of nerve damage, and sorbitol dehydrogenase inhibitors were employed to test this hypothesis. However, despite initially encouraging results, recent data show a lack of effect of sorbitol dehydrogenase inhibitors in preventing vascular, neurological and metabolic abnormalities in diabetic nerves.[44–46]

Protein kinase C Inhibitors (PKC)

Protein kinase C (PKC) is not a single enzyme but is a family of at least 12 enzymes that differ in their tissue distribution, mechanism of action and ability to phosphorylate certain substrates.[47] Each isoform has different functions and systems of regulation. In most cases, these enzymes are physiologically activated by phospholipid catabolites, such as diacylglycerol (DAG), and they phosphorylate Na^+K^+-ATPase, which has an important role in regulating nerve membrane potential.

Initial studies reported that total PKC activity was reduced in diabetic nerve, suggesting that the related reduced Na^+K^+-ATPase activation was responsible for nerve dysfunction.[48] However, recent evidence suggests a hyperglycemia-induced activation of PKC in nerve blood vessels. More specifically, the PKC-βII isoform is predominantly activated in the retina, kidney, heart and blood vessels of experimental diabetes, and its activation is associated with impaired endothelium-dependent vasodilation, decreased blood flow and ischemia.[49]

As a result of previous findings, the potential role of PKC inhibitors in preventing diabetic nerve damage is currently being investigated. A 2-week treatment with a non-specific inhibitor of PKC improved nerve blood flow and nerve conduction velocity in diabetic rats.[50] Moreover, these effects were mediated by an increase in endothelial nitric oxide synthesis (eNOS), rather than a restoration in Na^+K^+-ATPase activity, indicating a role of PKC in regulating eNOS activity. More recently, the effects of a PKC-β-selective inhibitor have also been explored in experimental diabetes. This specific isoenzyme inhibitor was as effective as an ARI in preventing nerve function delay and nerve blood flow impairment in diabetic rats.[51] As its effects were not related to changes in nerve total PKC activity, a selective effect on the vascular isoenzyme was strongly supported. Clinical trials are awaited to confirm the effectiveness and safety of these new compounds in human diabetes.

gamma-Linoleic Acid

gamma-Linoleic acid (GLA) is an essential fatty acid that is required for the production of arachidonic acid derivatives, such as prostaglandins. In experimental and human diabetes, a reduction in the hepatic Δ6-desaturation of linoleic acid, the main dietary source of omega6 essential acids, to GLA has been described This is believed to result in a reduction of nerve arachidonic acid content that reduces the synthesis of vasodilator prostanoids, such as prostaglandin (PG) analog PGE1, and leads to vasoconstriction. Several studies in experimental diabetes reported that GLA, in the form of a selected variety of evening primrose oil, was consistently effective in both preventing and reversing diabetic neuropathy.[52] The improvement in nerve blood flow and endoneurial oxygen tension was a constant finding.

As a result of the previous studies, GLA has been tested in human neuropathy for more than a decade. An initial 12-month clinical trial that explored the effects of a GLA treatment in mild human diabetic neuropathy indicated a beneficial effect.[53] However, subsequent trials failed to confirm these results and the use of GLA as a potential theurapeutic agent was abandoned.

Aminoguanidine

Another mechanism in the initiation of glucose-induced neurotoxicity is the non-enzymatic glycation of free amino groups in proteins that results in subsequent chemical rearrangements and the production of protein complexes known as Advanced glycation endproducts (AGE). Glucose itself can also undergo non-enzymatic auto-oxidation in a process that is closely interconnected with AGE formation. The excess formation of AGE is one of the major sources of oxidative stress in diabetes, since this process supplies reactive oxygen species. Furthermore, AGE react with their own specific receptor (RAGE), leading to overexpression of vascular cellular adhesion molecules that are related to endothelial dysfunction.

Over the last decade, a number of studies that used aminoguanidine, a potent inhibitor of AGE formation, documented its efficacy in blocking or slowing progression of neuropathy in experimental diabetes.[54,55] The aminoguanidine effects were accompanied by an improvement in nerve blood flow supporting a vascular protective effect of this compound, probably NO mediated as suggested by recent data.[56] However, contrary to the studies in rats, a recent study on diabetic baboons with established nerve damage showed that a 3-year treatment with aminoguanidine had no effect in restoring nerve conduction velocity and autonomic function in this primate model.[57] The role of aminoguanidine in human diabetes is still undetermined but additional clinical trials that aim to evaluate the effect of aminoguanidine in diabetic nephropathy are currently in progress.

Antioxidants

As mentioned earlier, mounting evidence suggests a close relationship between increased oxidative stress and the development of chronic complications in diabetes. Increased oxidative stress in diabetes results from increased generation of reactive oxygen species and/or diminished antioxidant defenses. Oxidative stress is believed to cause nerve damage via direct neurotoxic effects, through the promotion of neuronal apoptosis, and indirect neurotoxic effects, mainly by impairing the vasodilating action of NO.[58]

Several antioxidants have shown promising results in experimental neuropathy. α-Lipoic acid, the most powerful lipophilic antioxidant, was shown to be effective in improving nerve blood flow, nerve glucose uptake, myoinositol nerve content and sensory nerve conduction velocity.[59,60] In human diabetes, an initial clinical trial showed that a 3-week intravenous treatment with 600mg of α-lipoic acid significantly reduced various neuropathic symptoms, including pain, paresthesia and numbness.[61] However, these data were not confirmed in a subsequent study that evaluated the effect of intravenous treatment with 600mg/day of α-lipoic acid for 3 weeks followed by oral treatment (600mg three times a day) for 6 months in diabetic patients with symptomatic neuropathy.[62]

The effect of α-lipoic acid treatment on autonomic neuropathy has also been explored. In a multicenter trial, an oral dose of 800mg per day of α-lipoic acid for 4 months improved specific parameters of cardiac autonomic neuropathy compared to placebo.[63] Studies which will explore the effects of α-lipoic acid on both neuropathic symptoms and autonomic dysfunction, using more reliable outcome measures, are in progress. Therefore, until the results of these studies are reported, the use of α-lipoic acid in the treatment of symptomatic diabetic neuropathy cannot be recommended.

Neurotrophins

Neurotrophins are a family of soluble proteins that affect the differentiation, growth, maturation, function and survival of particular sets of neurons: the family includes NGF, BDNT, NT-3 and NT-4/5. Each of these factors is specifically trophic for different neuronal populations in the peripheral nervous system and this specificity is determined by the receptor expressed on the nerve fibers. NGF was the first neurotrophic factor to be identified and most of the available data are about this neurotrophin. NGF is retrogradely transported to the neuronal cell body, where it binds to a high-affinity receptor, tyrosine kinase A (TrKA), and a low-affinity receptor, p75, that are present in small unmyelinated fibers of sensory neurons and in sympathetic neurons of the autonomic nervous system.

In both experimental and human diabetes, NGF levels have been reported to be reduced. Furthermore, the action of NGF was also found to be defective as the expression of its high-affinity receptor TrKA is reduced.[64] Since NGF specifically supports small fiber sensory neurons and sympathetic neurons, its altered availability may impair the regeneration processes and, therefore, facilitate the progression of small nerve fiber degeneration.[65]

The potential of recombinant human NGF (rhNGF) as a putative treatment for small nerve fibers deficit in human diabetes has recently been examined. An initial 6-month phase II clinical trial reported that NGF, administered subcutaneously at the dose of 0.1μg/kg three times per week, was effective in ameliorating both objective and subjective indices of sensory damage compared to placebo.[66] However, a subsequent large multicenter 12-month phase III clinical trial,[67] which enrolled a large number of diabetic patients with sensory neuropathy, failed to confirm these findings, reporting that NGF treatment had no effect on small nerve fiber function. Further studies will be required before any firm conclusion regarding possible efficacy of the NGF can be drawn.

Vasodilators

Improvement of nerve blood flow may prove a key element in the therapy of diabetic neuropathy. A host of vasodilator compounds, including PG analogs PGE1 and PGI2, α-adrenoceptor blockers, angiotensin-converting enzyme (ACE) inhibitors and, to a lesser extent, calcium-channel antagonists, have been shown to prevent and/or reverse nerve damage in experimental diabetes.

In human disease, ACE inhibitors seem to be the most promising vasodilators, as they promote vasodilatation both by preventing the generation of the vasoconstrictor angiotensin II and improving the endothelial function.[68] Support for this hypothesis was offered by a recent single-center clinical trial that included diabetic patients with mild neuropathy, which showed that treatment with the ACE inhibitor trandolapril resulted in a modest improvement in peripheral nerve function.[69]

Further studies exploring the potential benefits of ACE inhibitors on human neuropathy are required before any final conclusions are reached.

New therapies for the treatment of painful diabetic neuropathy

Chronic painful diabetic neuropathy is a common, disabling and distressing problem that can affect a considerable number of diabetic patients. The etiology of the painful symptoms is poorly understood and its natural history is not clearly established. Nevertheless, a spontaneous remittance of the symptoms over a period of few months to 1 year should be expected in the majority of the affected patients.

Painful diabetic neuropathy has always been a therapeutic challenge to physicians and a number of algorithms have been proposed by different investigators. The main aim of these algorithms is symptomatic treatment and they usually consist of the stepwise introduction of different agents as well as non-pharmacological approaches. Steady improvement of the glycemic control, along with the introduction of simple analgesics, are usually the first steps in all algorithms and may be helpful in patients with mild symptomatology.

Topical capsaicin

Local application of capsaicin can be tried in case the glycemic control and analgesics fail to improve the symptoms. Capsaicin works by depleting substance P from peripheral sensory neurons, causing the treated area to become relatively insensitive to pain.[70] Capsaicin is applied four times a day over the affected areas and pain relief is usually seen within 14–28 days. Topical side effects include transient burning and skin irritation, but these usually diminish over time.

Tricyclic antidepressants

Tricyclic antidepressants, such as imipramine, amitryptiline and desipramine, are the most commonly used medications in large, well-conducted clinical trials and have been shown to be effective in reducing the severity of diabetic neuropathic pain.[71,72] They are usually administered once daily in small to moderate doses. Their side effects are sedation, urinary retention and orthostatic hypotension, which can limit their use considerably. Venlafaxine is a newer antidepressant agent that inhibits the re-uptake of serotonin, norepinephrine and dopamine, and also has a beneficial effect on painful neuropathy.[73,74] In comparison with previous antidepressants, it has the advantage that it does not block the muscarinic, histaminergic and adrenergic receptors, resulting in fewer side effects.

Anticonvulsants

Alternatives to antidepressants are the anticonvulsant drugs carbamazepine and gabapentin. Carbamazepine, although not tested on large numbers of diabetic patients, has been shown to decrease the intensity of neuropathic pain and has been considered a useful agent. In contrast, more data are available regarding gabapentin, structurally related to GABA neurotransmitter. Recent large clinical trials have showed that gabapentin at a dose of 900–3600mg/day improves not only the painful symptoms but also the associated sleep problems, the patient's mood and the quality of life.[75,76] As gabapentin has a very favorable side effect profile, it can be used as a first-line choice for the management of painful neuropathy.

Anti-arrhythmics

Anti-arrhythmic agents, such as lidocaine and oral mexiletine, have also been tried in painful neuropathy.[77] Mexiletine, when given in a dose that corresponds to the therapeutic dose interval of its anti-arrhythmic effect, reduces pain rapidly and can also promote a significant reduction in sleep disturbances. The drug is contraindicated for patients with conduction abnormalities and an ECG should be obtained before treatment.

Tramadol hydrochloride

Tramadol hydrochloride, a centrally acting synthetic, non-narcotic analgesic, has recently been shown to be effective and safe, providing long-term relief.[77,79] It binds to μ-opioid receptors and weakly inhibits norepinephrine and serotonin re-uptake. It has a low potential for abuse and a low incidence of anticholinergic side effects. Adverse effects include nausea, constipation, headache and somnolence. The dose can vary from 50 to 400mg/day.

Electrotherapy

In patients with severe symptoms that do not respond to pharmacologic agents, or the side effects preclude their use, electrotherapy, either transcutaneous or percutaneous, can be another option. Transcutaneous electrotherapy (TENS) has been reported to reduce diabetic neuropathic pain and discomfort with no side effects.[80,81] In addition, percutaneous electrical nerve stimulation (PENS) has also been shown to decrease pain, to improve physical activity, the sense of well-being and the quality of sleep, and to reduce the need for oral nonopioid analgesic medications.[82] These methods are currently recommended for very severe, non-responding cases by some authorities but, nevertheless, have not gained universal approval in daily clinical practice.

Advances in the treatment of diabetic autonomic neuropathy

The most recent advancements in the treatment of diabetic autonomic neuropathy are related to erectile dysfunction. Erectile dysfunction is defined as the inability to achieve and maintain an erection sufficient for satisfactory sexual intercourse with an estimated prevalence of greater than 30% in diabetic patients. Its etiology is multifactorial but autonomic neuropathy plays a major role. Until the advent of sildenafil, treatment options included external vacuum devices, intraurethral administration of alprostadil and intracavernosal injections of vasoactive drugs, as well as other therapies.

Sildenafil is a potent inhibitor of the cyclic guanosine monophosphate (cGMP)-specific phosphodiesterase type 5 (PDE5) in the corpus cavernosum and therefore increases the penile response to sexual stimulation. It is well tolerated and has conclusively been shown to be of benefit to diabetic males.[83,84] The recommended dose is 25–100mg taken $\frac{1}{2}$–4 hour before sexual activity. The most common adverse effects are headache, flushing, dyspepsia and visual disturbance. However, the physician should be aware that concurrent use of sildenafil and nitrate-containing drugs is contraindicated due to the potential for severe, potentially fatal hypotensive episodes.

Conclusions

Despite intensive efforts over that last two decades, little progress has been made in the treatment of diabetic neuropathy. However, as knowledge regarding the pathogenesis of the disease has greatly improved, it is hoped that this will result in the development of effective therapeutic interventions in the near future. The development of strategies that will combine various therapeutic agents, such as ARI, antioxidants and PKC inhibitors, offer the best possibility at present. It is hoped that more information about these efforts will become available over the next few years and that successful management of this condition will be developed.

References

1. American Diabetes Association, American Academy of Neurology. Consensus statement: report and recommendations of the San Antonio conference on diabetic neuropathy. Diabetes Care 1988; 11:592–7.

2. Dyck PJ, Kratz KM, Karnes JL, et al. The prevalence by staged severity of various types of diabetic neuropathy, retinopathy and nephropathy in a population-based cohort: the Rochester Diabetic Neuropathy Study. Neurology 1993; 43:817–24.

3. Young MJ, Boulton AJM, MacLeod AF, et al. A multicenter study of the prevalence of diabetic peripheral neuropathy in the United Kingdom hospital clinic population. Diabetologia 1993; 36:1–5.

4. Thomas PK. Classification, differential diagnosis and staging of diabetic peripheral neuropathy. Diabetes 1997; 46(Suppl 2): S54–S57.

5. Holzer SE, Camerota A, Martens L, et al. Costs and duration of care for lower extremity ulcers in patients with diabetes. Clin Ther 1998; 20:169–81.

6. Bird SJ, Brown SJ. The clinical spectrum of diabetic neuropathy. Semin Neurol 1996; 16:115–22.

7. Young MJ, Breddy JL, Veves A, Boulton AJ. The prediction of diabetic neuropathic foot ulceration using vibration perception thresholds. A prospective study. Diabetes Care 1994; 17:557–60.

8. Cavanagh PR, Imoneau GG, Ulbrecht JS. Ulceration, unsteadiness, and uncertainty: the biomechanical consequences of diabetes mellitus. J Biomech 1993; 26:23–40.

9. Veves A, Murray HJ, Young MJ, Boulton AJM. The risk of foot ulceration in diabetic patients with high foot pressure: a prospective study. Diabetologia 1992; 35: 660–3.

10. Pfeifer MA, Weinberg CR, Cook DL, et al. Correlations among autonomic, sensory, and motor neural function tests in untreated non-insulin-dependent diabetic individuals. Diabetes Care 1985; 8:576–84.

11. Rathmann W, Ziegler D, Jahnke M, et al. Mortality in diabetic patients with cardiovascular autonomic neuropathy. Diabet Med 1993; 10:820–4.

12. Stevens MJ, Feldman EL, Green DA. The aetiology of diabetic neuropathy: the combined roles of metabolic and vascular defects. Diabet Med 1995; 12:566–79.

13. Feldman EL, Stevens MJ, Green DA. Pathogenesis of diabetic neuropathy. Clin Neurosci 1997; 4:365–70.

14. Malik RA, Tesfaye S, Thompson SD, et al. Transperineurial capillary abnormalities in the sural nerve of patients with diabetic neuropathy. Microvasc Res 1994; 48:236–45.

15. Tooke JE. Possible pathophysiological mechanisms for diabetic angiopathy in Type 2 diabetes. J Diabetes Complic 2000; 14: 197–200.

16. Khan F, Elhadd TA, Greene SA, Belch JJ. Impaired skin microvascular function in children, adolescents, and young adults with Type 1 diabetes. Diabetes Care 2000; 23:215–20.

17. Veves A, Akbari CM, Primavera J, et al. Endothelial dysfunction and the expression of endothelial nitric oxide synthetase in diabetic neuropathy, vascular disease, and foot ulceration. Diabetes 1998; 47:457–63.

18. Feldman EL, Stevens MJ, Greene DA. Pathogenesis of diabetic neuropathy. Clin Neurosci 1997; 4:365–70.

19. Pham HT, Armstrong DG, Harvey C, et al. Screening techniques to identify the at risk patients for developing diabetic foot ulcers in a prospective multicentre trial. Diabetes Care 2000; 23:606–11.

20. Kennedy WR, Wendelschafer-Crabb G. Utility of skin biopsy in diabetic neuropathy. Semin Neurol 1996; 16:163–71.

21. Kennedy WR, Wendelschafer-Crabb G, Johnson T. Quantitation of epidermal nerves in diabetic neuropathy. Neurology 1996; 47:1042–8.

22. Hermann DN, Griffin JW, Hauer BS, et al. Epidermal nerve fiber density and sural nerve morphometry in peripheral neuropathies. Neurology 1999; 53:1634–40.

23. Hamdy O, Abou-Elenin A, LoGerfo FW, et al. Contribution of nerve-axon reflex-related vasodilation to the total skin vasodilation in diabetic patients with and without neuropathy. Diabetes Care 2001; 24:344–9.

24. Pirart J. Diabetes mellitus and its degenerative complications: a prospective study of 4400 patients observed between 1947 and 1973. Diabetes Care 1978; 1:168–88.

25. Diabetes Control and Complications Trial Research Group. The effect of intensive treatment of diabetes on the development and progression of long-term complications in insulin-dependent diabetes mellitus. New Engl J Med 1993; 329:977–86.

26. UK Prospective Diabetes Study Group. Intensive blood-glucose control with sulphonylureas or insulin compared with conventional treatment and risk of complications in patients with Type 2 diabetes (UKPDS 33). Lancet 1998; 352:837–53.

27. Diabetes Control and Complications Trial Research Group. The effect of intensive diabetes therapy on the development and progresion of diabetic neuropathy. Ann Intern Med 1995; 15:561–8.

28. Stratton IM, Adler AI, Neil HA, et al. Association of glycaemia with macrovascular and microvascular complications of Type 2 diabetes (UKPDS 35): prospective observational study. Br Med J 2000; 321:405–12.

29. Diabetes Control and Complications Trial Research Group. The absence of a glycemic threshold for the development of long-term complications: the perspective of the DCCT. Diabetes 1996; 45:1289–98.

30. Navarro X, Kennedy WR, Aeppli D, Sutherland DER. Neuropathy and mortality in diabetes: influence of pancreatic transplantation. Muscle Nerve 1996; 19:1009–16.

31. Kim J, Kyriazi H, Greene DA. Normalization of $Na^+–K^+$-ATPase activity in isolated membrane fraction from sciatic nerves of streptozotocin-induced diabetic rats by dietary myo-inositol supplementation in vivo or protein kinase C agonists in vitro. Diabetes 1991; 40:558–67.

32. Pfeifer MA, Schumer MP, Gelber DA. Aldose reductase inhibitors: the end of an era or the need for different trial designs? Diabetes 1997; 46(Suppl 2):S82–S89.

33. Nicolucci A, Carinci F, Graepel JG, et al. The efficacy of tolrestat in the treatment of diabetic peripheral neuropathy: a meta-analysis of individual patient data. Diabetes Care 1996; 19:1091–6.

34. Green DA, Arezzo JC, Brown MB, and the Zenarestat Study Group.

Effect of aldose reductase inhibition on nerve conduction and morphometry in diabetic neuropahty. Neurology 1999; 53: 580–91.

35. Hotta N, Sakamoto N, Shigeta Y, et al. Clinical investigation of epalrestat, an aldose reductase inhibitor, on diabetic neuropathy in Japan: multicenter study. Diabetic Neuropathy Study Group in Japan. J Diabetes Complic 1996; 10:168–72.

36. Yasuda H, Hirai H, Joko M, et al. Effect of aldose reductase inhibitor on cutaneous nerve fiber length in diabetic patients. Diabetes Care 2000; 23:705.

37. Mizuno K, Kato N, Makino M, et al. Continuous inhibition of excessive polyol pathway flux in peripheral nerves by aldose reductase inhibitor fidarestat leads to improvement of diabetic neuropathy. J Diabetes Complic 1999; 13:141–50.

38. Kato N, Mizuno K, Makino M, et al. Effects of 15-month aldose reductase inhibition with fidarestat on the experimental diabetic neuropathy in rats. Diabetes Res Clin Pract 2000; 50:77–85.

39. Cameron NE, Cotter MA. Impaired contraction and relaxation in aorta from streptozotocin-diabetic rats: role of the polyol pathway activity. Diabetologia 1992; 35:1011–19.

40. Stevens MJ, Dananberg J, Feldman EL, et al. The linked roles of nitric oxide, aldose reductase, and Na^+, K^+-ATPase in the slowing of nerve conduction in the streptozotocin diabetic rats. J Clin Invest 1994; 94:853–9.

41. Cameron NE, Cotter MA, Hohman TC. Interactions between essential fatty acid, prostanoid, polyol pathway and nitric oxide mechanisms in the neurovascular deficit of diabetic rats. Diabetologia 1996; 39:172–82.

42. Hamada Y, Nakamura J, Naruse K, et al. Epalrestat, an aldose reductase inhibitor, reduces the levels of N-(carboxymethyl)lysine protein adducts and their precursors in erythrocytes from diabetic patients. Diabetes Care 2000; 23:1539–44.

43. Ohi T, Saita K, Furukawa S, et al. Therapeutic effects of aldose reductase inhibitor on experimental diabetic neuropathy through synthesis/secretion of nerve growth factor. Expl Neurol 1998; 151: 215–20.

44. Titon RG, Chang K, Nyengaard JR, et al. Inhibition of sorbitol dehydrogenase. Effects on vascular and nerve dysfunction in streptozotocin-induced diabetic rats. Diabetes 1995; 44:234–42.

45. Cameron NE, Cotter MA, Basso M, Hohman TC. Comparison of the effects of inhibitors of aldose reductase and sorbitol dehydrogenase on neurovascular function, nerve conduction and tissue polyol pathway metabolites in streptozotocin-diabetic rats. Diabetologia 1997; 40:271–81.

46. Obrosova IG, Fathallah L, Lang HJ, Greene DA. Evaluation of a sorbitol dehydrogenase inhibitor on diabetic peripheral nerve metabolism: a prevention study. Diabetologia 1999; 42:1187–94.

47. Roberts RE, McLean WG. Protein kinase C isozyme expression in sciatic nerves and spinal cords of experimentally diabetic rats. Brain Res 1997; 754:147–56.

48. Kim J, Rushovich EH, Thomas TP, et al. Diminished specific activity of cytosolic protein kinase C in sciatic nerve of streptozotocin-induced diabetic rats and its correction by dietary myo-inositol. Diabetes 1991; 40:1545–54.

49. Koya D, King GL. Protein kinase C activation and the development

of diabetic complications. Diabetes 1998; 47:859–66.

50. Cameron NE, Cotter MA, Jack AM, et al. Protein kinase C effects on nerve function, perfusion, Na⁺K⁺-ATPase activity and glutathione content in diabetic rats. Diabetologia 1999; 42:1120–30.

51. Nakamura J, Kato K, Hamada Y, et al. A protein kinase C-beta selective inhibitor ameliorates neural dysfunction in streptozotocin-induced diabetic rats. Diabetes 1999; 48:2090–5.

52. Horrobin DF. Essential fatty acids in the management of impaired nerve function in diabetes. Diabetes 1997; 46(Suppl 2): S90–S93.

53. Keen H, Payan J, Allawi J, et al. Treatment of diabetic neuropathy with gamma-linolenic acid. The gamma-Linolenic Acid Multicenter Trial Group. Diabetes Care 1993; 16:8–15.

54. Sugimoto K, Yagihashi S. Effects of aminoguanidine on structural alterations of microvessels in peripheral nerve of streptozotocin diabetic rats. Microvasc Res 1997; 53:105–12.

55. Yagihashi S, Kamijo M, Baba M, et al. Effect of aminoguanidine on functional and structural abnormalities in peripheral nerve of STZ-induced diabetic rats. Diabetes 1992; 41: 47–52.

56. Cameron NE, Cotter MA. Rapid reversal by aminoguanidine of the neurovascular effects of diabetes in rats: modulation by nitric oxide synthase inhibition. Metabolism 1996; 45:1147–52.

57. Birrell AM, Heffernan SJ, Ansselin AD, et al. Functional and structural abnormalities in the nerves of Type I diabetic baboons: aminoguanidine treatment does not improve nerve function. Diabetologia 2000; 43:110–16.

58. Greene DA, Stevens MJ, Obrosova I, Feldman EL. Glucose-induced oxidative stress and programmed cell death in diabetic neuropathy. Eur J Pharmac 1999; 375:217–23.

59. Stevens MJ, Obrosova I, Cao X, et al. Effects of DL-alpha-lipoic acid on peripheral nerve conduction, blood flow, energy metabolism, and oxidative stress in experimental diabetic neuropathy. Diabetes 2000; 49:1006–15.

60. Kishi Y, Schmelzer JD, Yao JK, et al. Alpha-lipoic acid: effect on glucose uptake, sorbitol pathway, and energy metabolism in experimental diabetic neuropathy. Diabetes 1999; 48:2045–51.

61. Ziegler D, Hanefeld M, Ruhnau KJ, et al. Treatment of symptomatic diabetic peripheral neuropathy with the anti-oxidant alpha-lipoic acid. A 3-week multicentre randomized controlled trial (ALADIN Study). Diabetologia 1995; 38:1425–33.

62. Ziegler D, Schatz H, Conrad F, et al. Effects of treatment with the antioxidant alpha-lipoic acid on cardiac autonomic neuropathy in NIDDM patients. A 4-month randomized controlled multicenter trial (DEKAN Study). Deutsche Kardiale Autonome Neuropathie. Diabetes Care 1997; 20:369–73.

63. Tomlinson DR, Fernyhough P, Diemel LT. Role of neurotrophins in diabetic neuropathy and treatment with nerve growth factors. Diabetes 1997; 46(Suppl 2): S43–S49.

64. Malik RA. The pathology of human diabetic neuropathy. Diabetes 1997; 46(Suppl 2): S50–S53.

65. Apfel SC, Kessler JA, Adornato BT, et al. Recombinant human nerve growth factor in the treatment of diabetic polyneuropathy. NGF Study Group. Neurology 1998; 51:695–702.

66. Apfel SC, Schwartz S, Adornato BT, et al. Efficacy and safety of recombinant human nerve growth factor in patients with diabetic polyneuropathy: a randomized controlled trial. J Am Med Ass 2000; 284:2215–21.

67. Arcaro G, Zenere BM, Saggiani F, et al. ACE inhibitors improve endothelial function in Type 1 diabetic patients with normal arterial pressure and microalbuminuria. Diabetes Care 1999; 22:1536–42.

68. Malik RA, Williamson S, Abbott C, et al. Effect of angiotensin-converting-enzyme (ACE) inhibitor trandolapril on human diabetic neuropathy: randomised double-blind controlled trial. Lancet 1998; 352:1978–81.

69. Capsaicin Study Group. Treatment of painful diabetic neuropathy with topical capsaicin. Archs Intern Med 1991; 151:2225.

70. Kvinesdal B, Molin J, Froland A, Gram LF. Imipramine treatment of painful diabetic neuropathy. J Am Med Ass 1984; 251:1727.

71. Max MB, Lynch SA, Muir J, et al. Effects of desipramine, amitriptyline, and fluoxetine on pain in diabetic neuropathy. New Engl J Med 1992; 326:1250.

72. Davis JL. Painful peripheral diabetic neuropathy treated with Venlafaxine HCl extended release capsules. Diabetes Care 1999; 22:1909.

73. Lithner F. Venlafaxine in treatment of severe painful peripheral diabetic neuropathy. Diabetes Care 2000; 23:1710.

74. Backonja M, Beydoun A, Edwards KR, et al. Gabapentin for the symptomatic treatment of painful neuropathy in patients with diabetes mellitus. A randomized controlled trial. J Am Med Ass 1998; 280:1831.

75. Perez HET, Sanchez GF. Gabapentin therapy for diabetic neuropathic pain. Am J Med 2000; 108:689.

76. Oskarson P, Lins PE, Ljunggren JG. Efficacy and safety of mexiletine in the treatment of painful diabetic neuropathy. Diabetes Care 1997; 20:1594.

77. Harati Y, Gooch C, Swenson M, et al. Double-blind randomized trial of tramadol for the treatment of the pain of diabetic neuropathy. Neurology 1998; 50:1842.

78. Harati Y, Gooch C, Swenson M, et al. Maintenance of the long term effectiveness of tramadol in treatment of the pain of diabetic neuropathy. J Diabetes Complic 2000; 14:65–70.

79. Kumar D, Marshall HJ. Diabetic peripheral neuropathy: amelioration of pain with transcutaneous electrostimulation. Diabetes Care 1997; 20:1702.

80. Kumar D, Alvaro MS, Julka IS, Marshall HJ. Diabetic peripheral neuropathy: effectiveness of electrotherapy and amitriptyline for symptomatic relief. Diabetes Care 1998; 21:1322.

81. Hamza MA, White PF, Craig WF, et al. Percutaneous electrical nerve stimulation. A novel analgesic therapy for diabetic neuropathic pain. Diabetes Care 2000; 23:365.

82. Goldstein I, Lue TF, Padma-Nathan H, et al. Oral sildenafil in the treatment of erectile dysfunction. New Engl J Med 1998; 338:1397.

83. Price DE, Gingell JC, Gepi-Attee S, et al. Sildenafil: study of a novel oral treatment for erectile dysfunction in diabetic men. Diabet Med 1998; 15:821–5.

84. Rendell MS, Rajfer J, Wicker PA, et al. Sildenafil for treatment of erectile dysfunction in men with diabetes. J Am Med Ass 1999; 281:421.

85. Culebras A, Alio J, Herrera JL,

Lopez-Fraile MI. Effect of an aldose reductase inhibitor on diabetic peripheral neuropathy. Preliminary report. Arch Neurol 1981; 38:133–4.

86. Handelsman DJ, Turtle JR. Clinical trial of an aldose reductase inhibitor in diabetic neuropathy. Diabetes 1981; 30:459–64.

87. Fagius J, Jameson S. Effects of aldose reductase inhibitor treatment in diabetic polyneuropathy – a clinical and neurophysiological study. J Neurol Neurosurg Psychiatry 1981; 44:991–1001.

88. Judzewitsch RG, Jaspan JB, Polonsky KS, et al. Aldose reductase inhibition improves nerve conduction velocity in diabetic patients. New Engl J Med 1983; 308:119–25.

89. Jaspan J, Maselli R, Herold K, Bartkus C. Treatment of severely painful diabetic neuropathy with an aldose reductase inhibitor: relief of pain and improved somatic and autonomic nerve function. Lancet 1983; 2:758–62.

90. Young RJ, Ewing DJ, Clarke BF. A controlled trial of sorbinil, an aldose reductase inhibitor, in chronic painful diabetic neuropathy. Diabetes 1983; 32:938–42.

91. Lewin IG, O'Brien IA, Morgan MH, Corrall RJ. Clinical and neurophysiological studies with the aldose reductase inhibitor, sorbinil, in symptomatic diabetic neuropathy. Diabetologia 1984; 26:445–8.

92. Fagius J, Brattberg A, Jameson S, Berne C. Limited benefit of treatment of diabetic polyneuropathy with an aldose reductase inhibitor: a 24-week controlled trial. Diabetologia 1985; 28: 323–9.

93. O'Hare JP, Morgan MH, Alden P, et al. Aldose reductase inhibition in diabetic neuropathy: clinical and neurophysiological studies of one year's treatment with sorbinil. Diabet Med 1988; 5:537–42.

94. Guy RJ, Gilbey SG, Sheehy M, et al. Diabetic neuropathy in the upper limb and the effect of twelve months sorbinil treatment. Diabetologia 1988; 31:214–20.

95. Sima AA, Bril V, Nathaniel V, et al. Regeneration and repair of myelinated fibers in sural-nerve biopsy specimens from patients with diabetic neuropathy treated with sorbinil. New Engl J Med 1988; 319:548–55.

96. Ziegler D, Mayer P, Rathmann W, Gries FA. One-year treatment with the aldose reductase inhibitor, ponalrestat, in diabetic neuropathy. Diabetes Res Clin Pract 1991; 14:63–73.

97. Krentz AJ, Honigsberger L, Ellis SH, et al. A 12-month randomized controlled study of the aldose reductase inhibitor ponalrestat in patients with chronic symptomatic diabetic neuropathy. Diabet Med 1992; 9:463–8.

98. Ryder S, Sarokham B, Shand DG, Mullane JF. Human safety profile of tolrestat: an aldose reductase inhibitor. Drug Dev Res 1987; 11:131–43.

99. Boulton AJ, Levin S, Cornstock J. A multicentre trial of the aldose reductase inhibitor, tolrestat, in patients with symptomatic diabetic neuropathy. Diabetologia 1990; 33:431–7.

100. Macleod AF, Boulton AJ, Owens DR, et al. A multicentre trial of the aldose reductase inhibitor tolrestat, in patients with symptomatic diabetic peripheral neuropathy. North European Tolrestat Study Group. Diabetes Metab 1992; 18:14–20.

101. Santiago JV, Snksen PH, Boulton AJ, et al. Withdrawal of the aldose reductase inhibitor tolrestat in patients with diabetic neuropathy: effect on nerve function. The

Tolrestat Study Group. J Diabetes Complic 1993; 7:170–8.

102. Giugliano D, Marfella R, Quatraro A, et al. Tolrestat for mild diabetic neuropathy. A 52-week, randomized, placebo-controlled trial. Ann Intern Med 1993; 118:7–11.

103. Giugliano D, Acampora R, Marfella R, et al. Tolrestat in the primary prevention of diabetic neuropathy. Diabetes Care 1995; 18:536–41.

Index